OXFORD MEDICAL PUBLICATIONS

# Nutrition, diet, and oral health

# Nutrition, diet, and oral health

**Andrew J. Rugg-Gunn**

Professor of Preventive Dentistry and Honorary Consultant,
Department of Child Dental Health,
Director, WHO Collaborating Centre for Nutrition and Oral Health,
Co-Director, Human Nutrition Research Centre, Newcastle University

and

**June H. Nunn**

Senior Lecturer and Honorary Consultant
Department of Child Dental Health,
Newcastle University Dental School

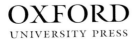

OXFORD
UNIVERSITY PRESS

# OXFORD
## UNIVERSITY PRESS

Great Clarendon Street, Oxford OX2 6DP

Oxford University Press is a department of the University of Oxford
and furthers the University's aim of excellence in research, scholarship,
and education by publishing worldwide in

Oxford New York

Athens Auckland Bangkok Bogotá Buenos Aires Calcutta
Cape Town Chennai Dar es Salaam Delhi Florence Hong Kong Istanbul
Karachi Kuala Lumpur Madrid Melbourne Mexico City Mumbai
Nairobi Paris São Paulo Singapore Taipei Tokyo Toronto Warsaw
and associated companies in Berlin Ibadan

Oxford is a registered trade mark of Oxford University Press

Published in the United States
by Oxford University Press Inc., New York

A catalogue record for this book is available from the British Library

Library of Congress Cataloging in Publication Data
Rugg-Gunn, A. J.
Nutrition, diet, and oral health / Andrew J. Rugg-Gunn and June H.
Nunn.
Includes index.
1. Nutrition and dental health. I. Nunn, June H. II. Title.
[DNLM: 1. Oral Health. 2. Dental Caries–prevention & control.
3. Nutrition. WU 113.7 R929n 1999]
RK281.R843 1999 617.6'01–dc21 99–11561

ISBN 0 19 262937 9

Typeset by EXPO Holdings, Malaysia

Printed in Hong Kong

# Preface

'We are what we eat'—and never before has there been such an emphasis on the way we are and what we eat. The general public has become increasingly aware of the link between diet and health; virtually every magazine you open has advice about diet and even the 'best seller' lists are dominated by books and videos from the latest fitness and diet guru. This is a welcome trend for oral health since good dietary practices are fundamental to the successful prevention of a variety of oral conditions. The intimate relationship between nutrition, diet, and oral health has become embedded in the teaching of undergraduate students, endorsed by the General Dental Council in their guidelines on the dental curriculum.

Our concept of a bad diet for those living in developed countries has changed considerably over the past 50 years: we are much more concerned with excesses of intake rather than deficiencies. Dental health education reflects this change and advice to curb excessive, frequent consumption of sugar is seen as much more relevant than concern about vitamin and mineral intake. Nevertheless, research indicates that teeth and other oral tissues are affected during their formation by nutrition, and that deficiencies can lead to malformations of tooth enamel which are aesthetically unacceptable and can increase susceptibility to disease. Not only can poor nutrition cause oral diseases but teeth, or rather lack of them, may influence nutrition. The incidence of cancer of the mouth is increasing and dietary factors are on both sides of the equation—causative and preventive.

The book first describes the effect of nutrients on the structure of teeth, followed by a summary of the ability of various components of diet to promote or prevent dental caries development. This is followed by a discussion of the erosive effect of diet, the effect of nutrition and diet on periodontal tissues and oral mucosa, and how lack of teeth affects food choice, nutrition, and health. This information is then brought together and advice for children and adults clarified. The final section of the book discusses the influences of government, industry, and other national and local bodies, and describes methods for improving the diet of patients. While each chapter is discrete, the practical relevance of this information is highlighted in numerous case reports. Evidence is often conveyed as figures or tables, and additional information is given in boxes. A small selection of material is suggested for further reading at the end of each chapter.

Many dental undergraduate courses in the UK and elsewhere have expanded their teaching of nutrition and this book should fill a gap in their reading list. The Department of Health has recommended close links between dentists, dietitians, and other health professions and this book has been written to assist this process.

*Newcastle upon Tyne*                                                     AJR-G
March 1999                                                                JHN

# Acknowledgements

We are grateful to a number of colleagues who have generously offered advice on the contents of this book; in particular we wish to mention Dr Paula Moynihan, Dr Anita Nolan, and Dr Neil Niven.

Editors of journals and other authorities have generously allowed us to use their material, and patients have agreed to publication of photographs; we acknowledge this support with thanks. The idea for this book came from Oxford University Press as a development of the textbook Nutrition and Dental Health: we are greatful to Oxford University Press for taking this forward in such a professional manner.

Inevitably, a project such as this eats into leisure time; we are both grateful to our families, especially Robert, William, Diane and Peter.

# Contents

# 1

# What it is all about

- Further reading

# What it is all about

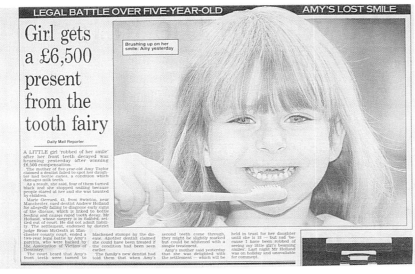

**Figure 1.1** Headlines from a national newspaper after dentist was sued for failure to diagnose 'bottle caries'.

*Girl gets a £6 500 present from the tooth fairy*
… So reads the headline in a national paper. The article goes on to describe how the parents of this seemingly lucky 5 year old sued the dentist because of his failure, allegedly, to diagnose the early signs of 'bottle caries'.

Most dentists in the UK work in general dental practice and the above case illustrates the importance of taking a careful history and giving the appropriate advice; a daily event for most of us. But dentists do not work in isolation—there is usually a dental team contributing to the care of patients. Members of the team are likely to be asked questions by patients or parents of young patients and expected not only to ask the right questions and give the right advice but also, importantly, to motivate patients to change their behaviour for the better. Our eating habits are moulded by many diverse influences and it is essential to understand these if advice is to be appropriate, accepted, and followed. The dentist and the dental team have to be aware of what influences behaviour in families, in communities, and indeed nationally. Knowing what advice is correct is important, and getting it right is one of the central themes of this book. But just giving advice, even correct advice, is unlikely to be enough. It has to be seen to be relevant to that patient for it to be accepted, and it has to be feasible for it to be followed.

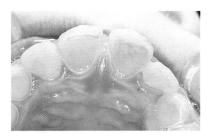

**Figure 1.2** Wear into dentine on the palatal surfaces of the permanent maxillary central incisor teeth.

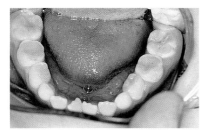

**Figure 1.3** Wear involving the occlusal surfaces of the mandibular primary molar teeth, especially the second primary molars.

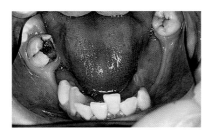

**Figure 1.4** The oral condition of Mr Briggs (case report): missing teeth, active decay, and fractured restorations.

## Case report

Laura is attending for a 6 monthly check-up. She is 10 years old and is fit and well and reports no symptoms. On examination, it is alarming to note how extensive the wear is on the palatal surfaces of her upper incisors (Fig. 1.2). Other teeth appear to be affected with some 'cupping' on the occlusal surfaces of her lower primary molar teeth (Fig. 1.3), but more advanced wear on the upper molar teeth. On questioning Laura and her mother, it seems that Laura's diet is to blame; her mother is at pains to point out how healthy the food is that Laura eats but it becomes obvious that even at this early age, Laura's new-found freedom at school means that she can choose what she eats at lunch: there is a drinks vending machine at school and she stops off at the corner shop with friends on the way to and from school ...

The cause of the erosion of teeth in the above case might be very clear but, at present, the lass is 'not fussed'. She is not in pain and her appearance is, as yet, unaltered. Why should she take your advice to cut down on fizzy drinks? To her, the alternatives you offer may not be acceptable. There are considerable pressures on her to continue—her own enjoyment, her peers, and advertising, as well as it having become a habit. A tough nut to crack. You will have to help her to devise a plan which will improve her dental health and be accepted.

Oral and dental health should not be isolated from general health, so it is important to ensure that your advice will not conflict with medical or dietetic advice and, indeed, general dental practitioners can do much to convey sound nutritional advice to improve health in general.

## Case report

Mr Briggs has gradually lost teeth over the years and has had a variety of partial dentures, mostly ill-fitting, because he will not see a dentist regularly. Sore spots mean that his dentures stay in the drawer most of the time and, as he now lives alone since his wife died, it does not terribly matter that he is without teeth for most of the time around the house. Eating is a problem though; he never did cook and he is not about to learn. Without many teeth, it is easier to have foods that require little or no chewing. In addition, getting out to shop is not so easy since he no longer drives and he finds it difficult to shop for fresh foods. It is sometimes just easier to have tea and toast or biscuits.

The reasons why this elderly man lost most of his teeth may be easy to establish but that is not his immediate concern. Lack of teeth and poor quality replacements for lost teeth have a strong influence on his choice of foods. Foods that are difficult to eat include fresh fruit and vegetables—and lack of these foods will put his general health at risk. Thus, there is a two-way interaction between nutrition, diet, and dental health. Incorrect diet causes dental diseases but, also, poor dental health can compromise healthy food choices and general health.

Bad teeth may not be the only barrier to improving dietary habits in the elderly. The price of foods, their availability close to home, and the amount of preparation of the foods in the home are all relevant. Fresh fruit and vegetables are heavy to carry home and may be more difficult to store and keep than other 'convenience' foods. The right advice is one thing, but achieving change is another. Your knowledge and skill will be required to bring about change, but you will find barriers to progress frequently in your path. Reducing these barriers is at the centre of health promotion, which is sometimes summarized as 'making healthy choices the easy choices'.

It is often useful to consider improving diet for oral health at three levels—the individual patient level, the community level, and the national level. The general dental practitioner, or primary dental care worker, obviously has an extremely important role in advising the individual patient. Community action can help to make healthy choices the easier choices, as shown in the following example.

## Case report

The oral health promotion unit of an urban area of Scotland decided to instigate a healthy eating policy by, first of all, having a health awareness week in local schools. This was specifically aimed at increasing the children's knowledge and acceptance of fruit and vegetables as part of their normal choice of school meals and beyond. An evaluation after the programme showed a change for the better, with more children choosing vegetables to accompany main meals and also choosing fruit as an alternative to puddings. These changes seem to have been sustained over 6 months.

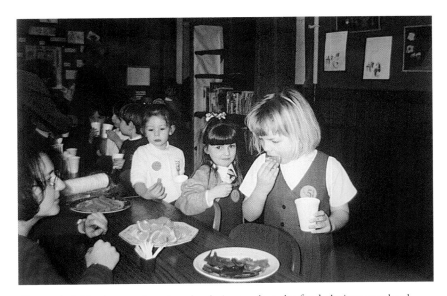

**Figure 1.5** Tasting sessions in school aim to alter the food choices at school meals in this healthy eating campaign in Scotland.

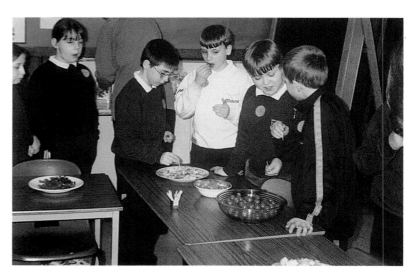

**Figure** 1.6 Allowing young people to sample different or rarely consumed foods aims to alter their food selection at school mealtimes.

Different types of dental personnel were included in this project. The general dental practitioner looked further than one-to-one advice with an individual patient and was able to answer questions generated by the project; the consultant in dental public health had an organizational role, liaising with her dietetic and educational colleagues; and the community dental officers and staff had an operational role.

Community health promotion programmes are important but often cannot tackle key issues such as television advertising, food labelling, approval of non-sugar sweeteners, or agricultural strategies and food subsidies. These have to be tackled nationally. Dentists need to be aware of how national regulations affect diet and oral health and how decisions about them can be influenced by the dental profession. It is difficult for a patient to heed your advice to reduce sugar consumption if foods are not labelled for sugar content in a user-friendly way.

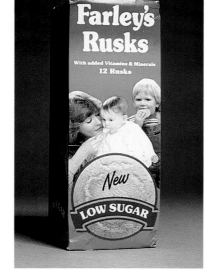

**Figure** 1.7 Consumers need to see at a glance if a product is likely to be 'dentally safe' from labelling that is not misleading.

## Case report

Take baby rusks for example; the one in Fig. 1.7 says 'low sugar', presumably compared with the ones next to it on the supermarket shelf. Manufacturers know that we are looking to see where 'sugar' is in the ranking of ingredients. Sucrose is reduced (so the product is lower in 'sugar') but other 'sugars' are added to compensate for taste—glucose syrup, for example. Individually, these sugars are present in much lower concentrations than the original sucrose so that the advertising claim above, with current labelling legislation in the UK, is legitimate. However, the total 'sugars' content is back up near the original amount it had been with sucrose alone! Manufacturers tend to sweeten such products to cater for mum's palate, not baby's who, if his palate was not bludgeoned with sweet-tasting foods and drinks, would not crave them to the extent that his mother may.

Improving diet is much more than just giving advice and we will consider these broader aspects of health promotion in Chapter 9.

So what oral diseases are diet-related? Although the prevalence and severity of dental caries have fallen in many countries, dental caries remains the most important diet-related oral disease (Fig. 1.8).

By the time of the 1993 UK Children's Dental Health survey, 30 per cent of those approaching school-leaving age had active decay and, for the first time, the prevalence of dental erosion was being recorded—over one half of 5–6 year olds and over one quarter of 14 year olds were affected (see Chapter 4).

Unchecked, dental caries causes infection and pain. It is expensive to treat and, a few years ago, was the second most expensive disease entity in the UK. Thus, it is still of social, medical, and economic importance. Appearance of teeth is important to social acceptability and unsightly teeth are an embarrassment (Figs 1.9 and 1.10).

Nutrition, diet, and oral health and disease are inextricably linked at all ages. Dentists and their dental team have a major role in preventing oral diseases, and can do much to improve general health through encouraging good dietary practices. To do this, you need to know the scientific basis for the advice, its relevance in each situation, the barriers and the motivation needed to achieve change. Your actions and advice need to be evidence-based—your patients will expect no less. The objective of this book is to provide you with the knowledge to do so.

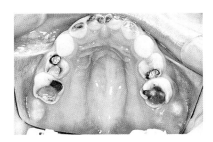

**Figure 1.8** Extensive dental decay in a 6 year old child—with a dietary cause.

## Dental caries

In the survey of oral conditions of pre-school children carried out in 1992–3 as part of the National Diet and Nutrition Survey, 17 per cent of toddlers had experience of dental decay. However, this average figure does not reflect wide variations depending on where you live—in Scotland this figure was 25 per cent, in the north of England 20 per cent, in Wales 19 per cent, and in the south of England 13 per cent. Children of unemployed parents had more decay experience, 22 per cent of children compared with 13 per cent of children whose parents were working. Likewise, for children with mothers who had 'A' level or higher qualifications, only 10 per cent of these children had experience of decay compared with 27 per cent of children whose mothers had no qualifications. These social inequalities must be taken into account when planning practical, personal and positive advice.

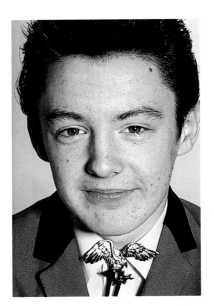

**Figure 1.9** This young man is apparently concerned about his appearance, as we see from the obvious attention he gives to his dress and hair; but he does not smile.

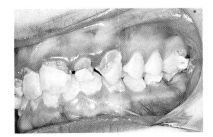

**Figure 1.10** This intraoral view of the person in Fig. 1.9 shows why he is not prepared to smile broadly—he sees how unsightly his teeth are and how they spoil his appearance.

## Periodontal disease

Scurvy used to be the scourge of sailors—bleeding gums and loosening of teeth being major symptoms. The addition of citrus fruits to the diets of sailors has become one of the landmarks of preventive medicine. Nutrients other than vitamin C affect the health of the periodontal tissues, which support teeth; this subject is considered in more detail in Chapter 5.

## Oral mucosa

The mouth has been termed the 'mirror of the body', with deficiency diseases affecting the appearance of the oral mucosa and tongue in particular. These are also discussed and the necessary investigations that need to be carried out for these patients given in Chapter 5.

## Defects of tooth structure

Poor nutrition is one of the more important of the many causes of defects in tooth structure. Of necessity, the nutritional insult has to occur during tooth formation, which effectively means before the age of 12 years. As the prevalence of caries falls, people are rightly more concerned that their teeth, especially the very visible front teeth, have an unblemished appearance. These front teeth are fully formed by about the age of 6 years. The important nutritional causes of developmental defects of enamel and what advice to give to minimize their occurrence are described in Chapter 2.

## Dental erosion

While defects of tooth structure are solely caused by insults during tooth formation, and dental caries is partly influenced by nutrition pre-eruptively but mainly by diet post-eruptively, erosion of teeth is a post-eruptive event. As yet, there is no evidence that pre-eruptive nutrition influences its occurrence. Dental erosion is a growing problem and its increasing prevalence is thought to be due to the very great rise in consumption of acidic soft drinks (Fig. 1.11). It is difficult and costly to treat and its prevention is being vigorously pursued—as shown in Chapter 4.

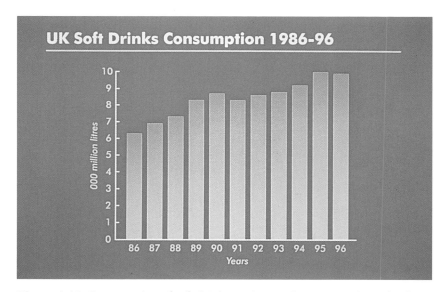

**Figure** 1.11 Consumption of soft drinks in the UK for the period 1986–96. Source: British Soft Drinks Association / Zenith International.

## Oral cancer

There are about 3 400 new cases of oral cancer per year in the UK, accounting for about 1 per cent of all new cases of cancers each year. On average, the 5 year survival rate for people with oral cancer in England and Wales is 50 per cent. With early detection this could be improved to 80 per cent. In part, that depends on those who see patients' mouths regularly—dentists—providing the right advice to prevent this disease which, unlike other forms of cancer, is largely due to lifestyle. It is becoming increasingly recognized that nutrition influences the occurrence of cancers in many situations, including the mouth. You can help your patient lessen the risk of oral cancer and also ensure adequate nutrition in those who have this debilitating disease. An important role for dentists is examining patients' mouths to detect oral cancer early when the chance of recovery is best.

## Ability to chew

The impact that a poor dentition has on food choice, nutrient intake, and general health has been touched on already. Although the example given was an elderly person, dentists need to be aware that lack of teeth can be a nutritional risk factor at any age. Unfortunately, it is all too common for young children to have many primary teeth extracted and these patients and their parents need advice on how and what to eat.

# Further reading

Buttriss, J. (ed.) (1994). *Nutrition in general practice. 1: Basic principles of nutrition*. The Royal College of General Practitioners, London.

Buttriss, J. (ed.) (1995). *Nutrition in general practice. 2: Promoting health and preventing disease*. The Royal College of General Practitioners, London.

# 2

# Nutrition and tooth development

# Nutrition and tooth development

In most societies now by far the most important role for good teeth is to enhance appearance. Facial appearance is tremendously important in determining an individual's integration into society. An essential component of any film star's face is a row of attractive, pearly white teeth. Unfortunately teeth are not always perfectly formed. There are many causes of these defects and this chapter describes how poor nutrition can cause defects of tooth structure and how this can be prevented.

In the first half of this century there was a strong belief that good nutrition, while teeth were forming, was the principal way to prevent dental caries. This was the age of the discovery of vitamins. We now know that the local topical effect of diet is a much more important cause of dental caries (see Chapter 3), but these early dental research workers were right to some extent, and how nutrition during tooth formation can influence the future caries susceptibility of teeth is described in this chapter.

## Tooth formation

Table 2.1 summarizes the times of tooth formation and eruption. The first signs of development of dental tissues occurs at around 28 days of intrauterine life and mineralization of the dentine and enamel of primary teeth begins at about 4–6 months *in utero*. Formation of enamel takes a long time and passes through a number of stages. These are the secretory phase, when the organic matrix is formed; the mineralization phase, which consists of crystal formation and crystal growth; and the maturation phase during which water and organic matter are withdrawn and the mineral content increases. Maturation of enamel is not fully complete until after the tooth has erupted into the mouth—a stage known as post-eruptive maturation. Thus, teeth may still be vulnerable to excess fluoride ingestion through late maturation, until about 7 years of age for many aesthetically important teeth—hence the need for caution in the use of fluorides before that age. For example, manufacturers of fluoride toothpastes will advise parents to supervise tooth-brushing, especially to limit the amount of fluoride dispensed from the tube, until this age, when a child can more readily spit excess toothpaste out.

## Case report

Janet had measles as a toddler: the impact on the developing dentition can be seen (Fig. 2.3) at the mid-incisal point of the upper central incisors, the incisal third of the lowers and the incisal edges of the maxillary lateral incisors and canines: hence the term chronological hypoplasia.

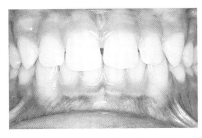

**Figure 2.1** Teeth of good quality and thus appearance.

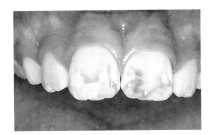

**Figure 2.2** Teeth of poor appearance because of extensive enamel opacities affecting the labial surfaces of the permanent maxillary incisor teeth.

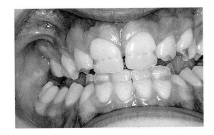

**Figure 2.3** Chronological hypoplasia affecting the maxillary and mandibular permanent teeth in a girl who had measles as a pre-school child.

Table 2.1.
## Chronology of development of the human dentition

| Tooth | | Enamel formation begins | Enamel completed | Eruption |
|---|---|---|---|---|
| **Primary dentition** | | (months *in utero*) | (months) | (months) |
| | Central incisor | 4 | 2 | 6 |
| | Lateral incisor | 4.5 | 2.5 | 8 |
| | Canine | 5 | 9 | 17 |
| | First molar | 5 | 6 | 13 |
| | Second molar | 6 | 11 | 24 |
| **Permanent dentition** | | (after birth) | (years) | (years) |
| | Central incisor | 3–4 months | 4–5 | 6–8 |
| | Lateral incisor | 3–12 months | 4–5 | 7–9 |
| | Canine | 4–5 months | 6–7 | 9–12 |
| | First premolar | 1.5–2 years | 5–6 | 10–12 |
| | Second premolar | 2–2.5 years | 6–7 | 10–12 |
| | First molar | At birth | 2.5–3 | 6–7 |
| | Second molar | 2.5–3 years | 7–8 | 11–13 |
| | Third molar | 7–10 years | 12–16 | 17–21 |

Based on Logan and Kronfeld (1933)

Enamel mineralization of permanent teeth is almost entirely postnatal. Sometimes the tips of the cusps of first permanent molars are mineralized by birth; certainly insults during the first 5 years of life can adversely affect the formation of these teeth.

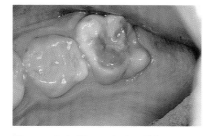

**Figure 2.4** Hypoplasia of the occlusal surface of this permanent maxillary first molar tooth as a consequence of a premature birth.

## Case report

John was born prematurely. The effect of this 'insult' can be seen on the teeth developing at the time, as hypoplastic defects, seen here (Fig. 2.4) on the occlusal surface of the maxillary first permanent molar.

Maxillary central incisors begin to mineralize soon after birth and this may be complete by 4–5 years; they usually erupt at 7–8 years. Therefore if the formation of these teeth is disturbed before about 5 years, their appearance might be damaged. As tooth formation begins near the incisal edge and works its way to the amelo-cemental junction, damage early in the first 5 years is more likely to affect the incisal area of the tooth and damage later will be more likely to affect the more cervical enamel.

## Types of defect

Defects of enamel formation can be divided into those in which the integrity of the enamel surface is maintained and those where the usual smooth enamel surface is interrupted by pits, lines, or larger areas of missing enamel. Several terms have been used to describe these defects—opacities, mottling, hypoplasia—and sometimes 'dental fluorosis' is used on the assumption that excessive ingestion of fluoride has been the cause.

A widely used index for classifying these defects has been proposed by the World Health Organization (WHO) and the Fédération Dentaire Internationale (FDI), called the 'developmental defects of enamel' (DDE) index. This index differentiates between defects which are 'diffuse' (Fig. 2.5), 'demarcated' (Fig. 2.6), and 'hypoplastic' (Fig. 2.7).

# Causes of dental enamel defects

Poor nutrition is only one of the many causes of dental enamel defects. Causes can be localized, such as a blow to a primary incisor (perhaps due to a toddler falling whilst learning to walk) resulting in damage to the forming permanent incisor. General causes are more common and the broad headings of these are given in Table 2.2. Those with a nutritional component are shown in bold and will be considered in turn.

## Linear enamel hypoplasia of primary teeth

### Case report

Figure 2.8 shows the teeth of a young boy who is one of 13 children of a destitute family living in an urban slum in a developing country. The family were reliant on aid to provide their most basic needs and his early years have been marred by diarrhoeal episodes and severe gastrointestinal upsets.

Linear enamel hypoplasia (LEH) is a well recognized defect of dental development in children living in communities in which malnutrition is widespread. The lesion is characterized by a horizontal groove most frequently found on the labial surfaces of primary incisors, affecting enamel formed during the neonatal period. The defects become stained soon after eruption and these teeth seem especially prone to develop dental caries, often being reduced to black stumps.

## Deficiencies of vitamin D, calcium and phosphorus, and enamel hypoplasia

Vitamin D is intimately involved with calcium metabolism and calcification, and it is not surprising that there has been considerable interest in its role in tooth formation. The story goes back 90 years, to 1918, when a remarkable woman—Lady May Mellanby—reported that dogs reared on a diet deficient in a 'fat soluble A accessory food factor' (which she subsequently recognized as vitamin D) had delayed development of teeth, which had very deficient, poorly calcified enamel. She carefully examined children's teeth, both in the mouth and under the microscope, and concluded that many teeth were hypoplastic and this

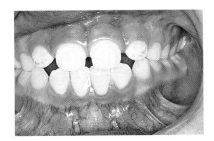
**Figure 2.5** Diffuse enamel opacities affecting almost the entire labial surface of these maxillary incisor teeth.

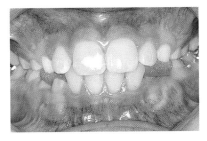
**Figure 2.6** Demarcated opacities—well circumscribed and demarcated from the surrounding normal enamel on the incisal half of the labial surface of the upper right permanent maxillary central incisor tooth (tooth 11).

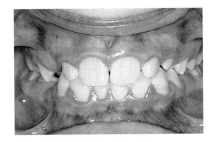
**Figure 2.7** Hypoplastic pits involving most of the labial surface of the permanent maxillary central incisor teeth.

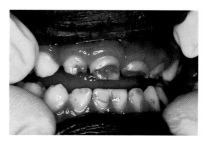

**Figure 2.8** Dental caries superimposed on linear enamel hypoplasia of primary maxillary incisor teeth.

Table 2.2.
A classification of the most common causes of developmental defects of dental enamel

SYSTEMIC CAUSES

| | |
|---|---|
| Genetically determined | Amelogenesis imperfecta |
| Chromosomal abnormalities | Trisomy 21 |
| Congenital defects | Heart disease |
| Inborn errors of metabolism | Phenylketonuria |
| **Neonatal disturbances** | Premature birth |
| | **Hypocalcaemia** |
| | Haemolytic anaemia |
| Infectious diseases | Rubella |
| Allergies | Asthma |
| Neurological disturbances | Tuberous sclerosis |
| **Endocrinopathies** | **Hypoparathyroidism** |
| | **Diabetes mellitus** |
| **Nutritional deficiencies** | **Vitamins** |
| | **Protein** |
| | **Energy** |
| | **Minerals** |
| Nephropathies | Nephrotic syndrome |
| **Enteropathies** | **Non-specific diarrhoea** |
| | **Coeliac disease** |
| **Intoxications** | Tetracyclines |
| | **Vitamin D** |
| | **Fluoride** |
| | **Other minerals** |

LOCAL CAUSES

| | |
|---|---|
| Trauma | Falls |
| | Surgery |
| Irradiation | Radiotherapy |
| Local infection | Periapical infections of primary teeth |

Nutritionally related causes are in bold. Based on Pindborg (1982)

was caused by vitamin D deficiency. She noticed that the appearance of children's teeth improved between 1929 and 1943 and attributed this to an improved diet, notably the introduction of cheap milk in 1934 and of the provision of cod liver oil to pregnant and lactating mothers, infants, and young children and the addition of vitamins A and D to margarine and calcium carbonate to bread. Fewer hypoplastic teeth were observed in children attending private schools in London compared with state run schools, which strengthened Mellanby's view that nutrition influenced the occurrence of hypoplastic teeth.

An explanation for the way nutrition may cause enamel hypoplasia was presented by Nikiforuk and Fraser in 1981. They labelled it a 'unifying concept' for the aetiology of enamel hypoplasia. Their study involved the thorough examination of 56 patients in Toronto, Canada, over 25 years. Ten of these patients had hereditary vitamin D dependency rickets—they had severe rickets, low plasma calcium and inorganic phosphorus, and all had hypoplastic teeth. Twenty-five patients had X-linked hypophosphataemia—they had rickets, low plasma inorganic phosphorus but normal plasma calcium, and well formed teeth without hypoplasia. The 21 patients with hypoparathyroid/pseudohypoparathyroid conditions had no rickets, high plasma phosphorus but low plasma calcium—15 of these had hypoplastic teeth. Thus, enamel hypoplasia only occurred in children with hypocalcaemia and no relation was found between enamel hypoplasia and plasma phosphorus levels. They also suggested that hypocalcaemia was the mechanism by which chronic diarrhoea caused dental hypoplasia.

The importance of the role of vitamin D and plasma calcium levels in the aetiology and prevention of enamel hypoplasia was illustrated by the results of a randomized clinical trial in Edinburgh. Five hundred and six pregnant women received vitamin D supplements from the 12th week of pregnancy and they were compared with 633 'control' pregnant women who did not receive a supplement. Both mothers who received the supplement and their infants had higher plasma concentrations of calcium than did the 'control' mothers and infants. When the teeth of the infants were examined in their third year, the occurrence of hypoplasia was very much lower in the 'supplemented' group than in the 'control' group.

## Fluoride and defects of dental development

The appropriate use of fluorides has been the most important method of controlling caries and is likely to be of great benefit for some time to come. These benefits will be discussed later in this chapter and in Chapter 3. The disadvantage of fluoride is that excessive ingestion causes developmental defects of enamel.

## Case report

Lucy's teeth (Fig. 2.9) illustrate the problem caused by ingestion of an adult concentration (1450 ppm) fluoride toothpaste. She was also taking a daily fluoride dietary supplement. The appearance of these diffuse opacities improved with time and there was no request for any treatment, despite the fact that one of the parents was a plastic surgeon!

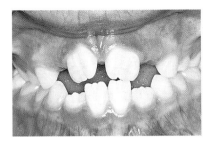

**Figure 2.9** Diffuse enamel opacities affecting the erupted permanent teeth, probably as a consequence of ingestion of high concentration fluoride toothpaste concurrently with a fluoride supplement, during the pre-school years.

The link between excessive fluoride ingestion and unsightly teeth goes back 100 years. The classical epidemiological studies which unravelled the relationship between dental opacities, fluoride ingestion, and dental caries began when a young American dentist left dental school in Pennsylvania to practise in the southern states of America where he was surprised to see that the teeth of most of his patients had severe intrinsic discoloration which he called 'Colorado stain'. Observation of the geographical distribution of the stain linked its occurrence to

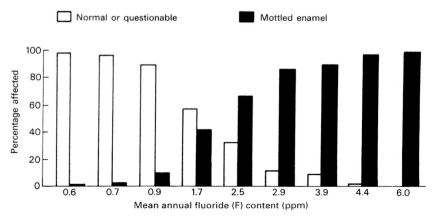

Figure 2.10 The prevalence of mottled enamel in areas with differing concentrations of fluoride in the water supply. Source: Dean (1936).

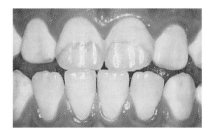

Figure 2.11 A child with amelogenesis imperfecta. Compare with Figure 2.12. (Reproduced with permission of Professor GB Winter.)

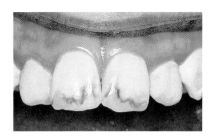

Figure 2.12 Diffuse enamel opacities affecting the erupted permanent teeth, probably as a consequence of 'eating' high concentration fluoride toothpaste as a pre-school child.

the water supplies of those localities and it was found subsequently that high concentrations of fluoride were responsible (Fig. 2.10). Later, it was also appreciated that dental caries experience was lower in areas with moderate concentrations of fluoride in water supplies than in areas with low concentrations of fluoride.

There has been much debate about whether the cause of an enamel defect can be determined from the appearance of the defect. With some non-nutritional causes, such as ingestion of tetracycline drugs, the cause is quite clear from the appearance. While excessive fluoride ingestion is undoubtedly an important cause of enamel opacities, and some indices for describing these defects have been labelled 'fluorosis indices', many people believe that it is not possible to be certain that excessive fluoride ingestion was the cause purely from appearance.

Figure 2.11 illustrates the mouth of a child who has amelogenesis imperfecta whilst Fig. 2.12 shows the mouth of a child with diffuse white/brown opacities as a consequence of 'eating' fluoride toothpaste as a toddler. This case shows the importance of taking a careful history in order to reach a diagnosis on the most likely cause (Boxes 2.1 and 2.2).

It now seems that there can be interactions between different causes of enamel opacities so that the defects are more pronounced than you might expect from any single cause. This can be illustrated by three examples, all of which involve fluoride ingestion.

The first example comes from New Zealand. This is a country with a high standard of nutrition. Over 1000 children born in Dunedin in 1972 were monitored closely every 2 years. The presence of dental enamel defects in permanent teeth was compared with relevant medical and dental histories. Overall, exposure to fluoride affected prevalence but the only two other factors to be significantly related to the occurrence of enamel hypoplasia were chicken-pox before the age of 3 years and trauma to deciduous incisors. Asthma was also a risk factor but only in areas with moderate levels of fluoride in water supplies and not in areas with low levels of fluoride in water supplies.

Box 2.1  **Questions to ask**

Was the pregnancy and birth uneventful?

Has the child had any major systemic upsets during the period of development of the affected teeth?

Did the child need frequent medication during the period of development of the affected teeth?

Where has the child lived—fluoride or non-fluoride areas?

Is there any family history of defects affecting the teeth?

What were the first (baby or milk) teeth like? (if shed already)

At what age did tooth-brushing start?

Was toothpaste used at this stage and if so, what type and how much?

Who did the tooth-brushing as a toddler? Parents or toddler, or both?

Did the child like toothpaste, for example did they suck it off the brush and/or help themselves to toothpaste?

Box 2.2  **Points to consider on examination**

Are the teeth sensitive?

Are all teeth affected, but at different stages of development?

Does the enamel appear to be missing in significant quantities?

Does the enamel feel soft to probing?

Do the tooth surfaces in occlusion appear worn?

Does the radiographic appearance suggest normal or deficient enamel, with or without other features, for example, taurodontism?

The second example comes from Saudi Arabia (Fig. 2.13) where there is moderate malnutrition. Excessive concentrations of fluoride in water and malnutrition were both risk factors and they had an additive effect. This study also showed that respiratory diseases (such as asthma) and enteropathies (such as coeliac disease) were risk factors in an area with moderate water fluoride levels, in agreement with other reports from Australia and Sweden.

The third example comes from Africa and is the most difficult to understand. The African Rift Valley contains areas with very high levels of fluoride in water (up to 20 mg F/l) and dental opacities are universal and severe. One unexpected finding was that the prevalence and severity of opacities increased with increasing altitude, leading to speculation that hypoxia might be a risk factor. Subsequent work in America and Sweden has shown, in rat experiments, that both fluoride and hypoxia are risk factors for enamel opacities. It does seem as if disturbance of the acid–base balance in plasma—as is likely to occur with altitude and maybe in premature births and asthma—as well as malabsorption of nutrients—as occurs

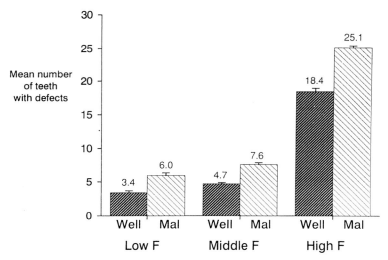

**Figure** 2.13 Mean number of teeth with developmental defects of enamel for well (Well) and malnourished (Mal) boys in the three regions of Saudi Arabia. Source: Rugg-Gunn *et al.* (1997).

in coeliac disease, vitamin D deficiency, non-specific diarrhoea, and general nutrition—may be risk factors for the development of enamel opacities.

From the above discussions it should be clear that there are many causes of developmental defects of enamel, some of which are related to nutrition. The most important cause of these nutritionally related defects is fluoride, and the concentration of fluoride in water is very clearly positively related to the prevalence and severity of enamel defects. These are defects caused by an excess of a nutrient (fluoride); excess of some other trace elements can also cause defects although their public health significance is likely to be tiny compared with that of fluoride. Nutritional deficiencies are also clearly causes of defects of enamel formation, probably through a variety of mechanisms. It would seem that plasma calcium level is important, with hypocalcaemia a clear risk factor. Plasma acid–base balance also would appear to be important but the exact mechanism and its possible link with plasma calcium levels have yet to be established.

# Nutrition during tooth development and caries risk

Can nutrition during tooth development influence future caries susceptibility? The answer is—yes it can—but this effect is relatively small compared with the local intraoral effect of diet. The local intraoral effect of diet is discussed in detail in Chapters 3 and 4.

The first half of this century was the age of discovery of deficiency diseases—the vitamin era—and caries was considered primarily to be a deficiency disease. In the years following the Second World War, advice about eating often urged mothers to give their young children diets rich in calcium and vitamin D so that they would form strong healthy bones and teeth: the inference was that these strong teeth would be less likely to decay. Although this is sound advice as far as the skeleton is concerned, there has always been little evidence to substantiate the view that good nutrition early in life helps to prevent dental decay by a systemic effect. This certainly does not mean that good nutrition should be discouraged, it merely reflects the current view that, in developed countries, diet has a much greater effect locally in the mouth on erupted teeth than it does pre-eruptively while the teeth are still forming. Indeed, the Health Education Authority in the UK stopped giving advice concerning calcium, vitamin D, and strong healthy teeth many years ago, in order to concentrate the dietary aspect of dental health education on two uncontroversial messages: reduce sugar consumption and drink optimally fluoridated water. It should be emphasized that these remarks concerning the unimportance of nutrition (other than fluoride) while teeth are forming apply at the present time to developed countries where standards of nutrition are generally adequate—the same may not apply in countries where severe malnutrition is prevalent.

The worldwide variation in the severity of dental caries has changed in recent years with a marked fall in the incidence of dental caries in many developed countries (which is almost certainly due to the widespread use of fluorides), and the rise in dental caries in many developing countries paralleling a rise in sugar consumption. However, where sugar is available in developing countries, the severity of dental caries seems to be higher than would be expected from experience in developed countries, especially in the deciduous dentition, which has led a number of people to ask whether malnutrition may enhance the cariogenic effect of fairly modest levels of sugar in the diet.

## Vitamin D

It is worth reminding ourselves that 96 per cent of dental enamel is apatite mineral—principally calcium and phosphorus—and that vitamin D is intimately related to calcium metabolism. Earlier in this chapter, the work of Lady May Mellanby was discussed. She showed that vitamin D deficiency led to hypoplastic teeth in dogs and suggested that this also occurred in humans. She then suggested that these hypoplastic teeth were more susceptible to caries, from her observation that carious teeth were more often hypoplastic than would be expected by chance. Lady Mellanby then began a series of clinical trials in the 1930s which indicated that dietary supplements of vitamin D (such as cod liver oil) resulted in decreased caries development in children. In one trial, the two comparative groups of children received supplements of olive oil (low in vitamin D) or treacle. It is surprising that Lady Mellanby's views of the importance of vitamin D in protecting against dental caries did not get more support. In fairness, the very important, costly, and influential Vipeholm study on diet and caries conducted in Sweden between 1946 and 1951 incorporated a 'vitamin period' into its plan. The influence of the vitamin and bone meal supplements was negligible compared with the tremendous effect of the later sugar supplementations. However, these subjects were adults whose teeth were fully formed.

## Box 2.3 Nutrition and tooth development

Enamel defects
 – inherited
 – acquired
Nutritional risk factors
 – vitamin D
 – calcium
 – phosphorus
 – fluoride
 – malnutrition

Since the Mellanby period, there have been a few reports which have kept alive the view that vitamin D may have some influence on caries development. Some schools in Canada have installed 'full spectrum' lighting (with high ultra-violet output) in classrooms. Children exposed to this light were found to have lower caries increment over 2 years than children attending classrooms with conventional lighting. In England, caries development was inversely related to dietary vitamin D intake, even when the data were standardized on possible confounding factors. An unexplained feature of this study was that this statistically highly significant result was found only in boys and not in girls.

## Calcium and phosphorus

'Does hardness of water affect the occurrence of disease?' This has been an interesting question for many years. There is some evidence that it affects the prevalence of coronary heart disease but does it affect dental health? There are four reports of epidemiological studies—one in South Africa and three in the USA—which lend support to the view that caries is inversely related to hardness of water. However, this relationship is fairly weak and certainly considerably weaker than the inverse relationship between water fluoride concentration and dental caries prevalence.

## Fluoride

In the 1950s and 1960s, caries experience was very high in many developed countries. Since then, it has declined dramatically to a moderate level. This welcome improvement coincided with the widespread introduction of fluoride into toothpastes and, in some countries, into other vehicles. This has been a great success story in the prevention of dental caries. Fluoride can act in two ways—the pre-eruptive effect, while teeth are forming, and the post-eruptive intraoral effect. It used to be thought that the pre-eruptive effect was the more important—incorporating fluoride into the forming tooth. However, it is now quite clear that the local intraoral (post-eruptive) effect of fluoride is more important and this latter aspect will be considered under 'protective factors' in Chapter 3. There is an opinion that the pre-eruptive influence of fluoride is negligible, but this is a minority view and the evidence does not support it. The great advantage of fluoride is that it prevents caries in a variety of ways, one of which is by being incorporated into forming enamel as fluorapatite, which is less soluble than the more common hydroxyapatite.

The most thorough investigation of the relative importance of pre-eruptive fluoride was undertaken in the Netherlands using data from the very well conducted Tiel and Culumborg water fluoridation study. The water supplies of Tiel were fluoridated from 1953 to 1973; Culumborg was the control town. Using epidemiological data collected before, during, and for some time after this period, it was possible to dissect out the caries reduction due to the pre-eruptive fluoride exposure alone, post-eruptive fluoride exposure alone, and both pre- and post-eruptive fluoride exposure. The pre-eruptive effect was substantial. In other words adequate but not excessive ingestion of fluoride during tooth formation is beneficial in caries prevention. However, it is also true to say that continued intraoral exposure to fluoride is essential for continued caries prevention throughout life. Many fluoride vehicles are made for local intraoral effect only—toothpastes and mouth-rinses are examples—and have been highly effective. Others, for example water, salt, and dietary supplements, provide both pre-eruptive and post-eruptive effects.

Because of the phenomenal success of fluoride in preventing dental caries, other trace elements have been examined closely. The heyday for this research was in the 1950s and 1960s when methods of detecting low concentrations of elements became simpler and more accurate. Molybdenum and strontium are caries-preventive elements—evidence coming from epidemiological and animal studies. Lithium may also be caries-preventive but evidence is confined to epidemiological studies. Selenium tends to be associated with an increase in caries but evidence is equivocal. Overall, only fluoride is of practical significance.

## Maximizing nutrition during tooth development for healthy teeth

Malnutrition in infancy and childhood affects tooth formation. Malnutrition is commonly due to energy deficiency and/or protein deficiency, but it is very possible that other nutrients are deficient as well. The underlying mechanism, as far as tooth development is concerned, would seem to be hypocalcaemia and

**Box 2.4 Key points—fluoride**

- Very effective in caries prevention
- Acts in a variety of ways
- Its local intra-oral action is very important
- Fluoride ingestion confers some systemic benefits.

Table 2.3.
Recommended fluoride intake for prophylaxis against caries

| Age | Agent | Caries risk | |
|---|---|---|---|
| | | Low risk | High risk |
| 6 months–3 years | Fluoride supplements | — | 0.25 mg F/day |
| | F toothpaste | 600 ppm F | 600–1000 ppm F |
| | Professionally applied fluorides | — | 3–4 times per year |
| | Home F rinsing | — | Not recommended |
| 3–6 years | Fluoride supplements | — | 0.5 mg F/day |
| | F toothpaste | 600 ppm F | 600–1000 ppm F |
| | Professionally applied fluorides | — | 3–4 times per year |
| | Home F rinsing | — | Not recommended |
| 6+ years | Fluoride supplements | — | 1.0 mg F/day |
| | F toothpaste | 1000–1500 ppm F | 1000–1500 ppm F |
| | Professionally applied fluorides | — | 3–4 times per year |
| | Home F rinsing | — | Daily |

*Note*: Patients may change risk category, thus it is important to re-assess risk at regular intervals with diet enquiries and bitewing radiographs as well as clinical examination.

disturbance of plasma acid–base balance. There has been sporadic evidence that vitamin D is important in preventing enamel hypoplasia and maybe dental caries, and there is some evidence that water hardness is inversely related to caries development. It is assumed that the effect is pre-eruptive, but this has not been clearly established.

## Summary

- By far the biggest nutritional influence on development of enamel and subsequently dental caries is fluoride. Most of fluoride's beneficial effect is post-eruptive, but it does also have a pre-eruptive caries-preventive effect.

- Excessive fluoride ingestion is one of the major causes of developmental defects of enamel and the dental team has a responsibility for advising patients how to maximize the beneficial effects of fluoride while minimizing the risks of causing enamel defects—this will be considered again in Chapter 7.

- Many communities throughout the world ingest excessive amounts of fluoride from drinking waters which contain too much fluoride. Defluoridation of water supplies has been practised in the USA, India, East Africa, and Thailand. The simplest method is to change water supply to one containing less fluoride, but that option is usually not available.

- The most common method is to filter water through material which will absorb fluoride. These materials include hydroxyapatite, bone char, activated carbon, lime, and alum. Ion exchange resins have also been used but are expensive. The most successful defluoridation plants have been in the USA, leading to substantial falls in the prevalence of dental fluorosis. Successful schemes in Asia and Africa have tended to use household filters, rather than defluoridation plants linked to public water supplies.

- In many countries, the problem of fluorosis has increased as villages change from using surface water (e.g. rivers) to bore wells, for hygiene reasons, since the water from bore wells contains a higher concentration of fluoride than does surface water.

## Further reading

Cockburn, F., Belton, N. R., Purvis, R. J., Giles, M. M., Brown, J. K., Turner, T. L. *et al.* (1980). Maternal vitamin D intake and mineral metabolism in mothers and their newborn infants. *Br. Med. J.* ii, 11–14.

Nikiforuk, G. and Fraser, D. (1981). The aetiology of hypoplasia: a unifying concept. *J. Pediatr.* **98**, 888–93.

Pindborg, J. J. (1982). Aetiology of developmental enamel defects not related to fluorosis. *Int. Dent. J.* **32**, 123–34.

Rugg-Gunn, A. J. (1993). *Nutrition and dental health*, Chapters 2–4. Oxford University Press, Oxford.

Winter, G. B. (1996). Amelogenesis imperfecta with enamel opacities and taurodontism: an alternative diagnosis for 'idiopathic dental fluorosis'. *Br. Dent. J.* **181**, 167–72.

# Diet and dental caries

# Diet and dental caries

## Introduction

In 1950, a report by an American research group—Kite and his colleagues—was published, which demonstrated very clearly that dental caries was caused by the presence of food in the mouth. In their experiments, rats were fed adequate amounts of a cariogenic diet, but half of the rats were fed this diet by stomach tube (thereby bypassing the mouth) and the other half of the rats fed in the usual way. Dental caries only occurred in the rats who fed in the usual way and no caries occurred in the rats fed by stomach tube (Table 3.1). In the same series of experiments, Kite also investigated the effect of removing major salivary glands on caries development. Caries experience was much greater in the desalivated rats—but again only in the rats which fed in the usual way (Table 3.1)—demonstrating the important role of saliva in caries prevention.

Four years later, another key study was published, also in America, by Orland and colleagues. They had developed a system for rearing rats under germ-free conditions. When these rats were fed a cariogenic diet, dental caries did not develop, in contrast to similar rats fed the same diet but not reared in germ-free conditions and allowed to acquire the usual mixed microbial flora (Table 3.2).

These experiments have been replicated, and demonstrate clearly that food in the mouth and the presence of microorganisms are essential for caries development. For the third important aspect to understanding caries development we need to look back over 100 years to the pioneering work of Miller, an American working in Berlin. He showed that carbohydrate-containing foods (but not meat), when incubated with saliva, caused demineralization of teeth *in vitro*. Further progress on the 'acidogenic theory of caries aetiology' had to wait until the development of microelectrodes capable of measuring pH in dental plaque— this work was pioneered by Stephan in the 1940s. He showed that the resting

Table 3.1.
The mean number of carious lesions in rats fed a cariogenic diet, either conventionally or by stomach tube, for rats with and without salivary glands

| Salivary glands | Conventional | Tube-fed |
|---|---|---|
| Intact | 6.7 | 0 |
| Desalivated | 28.8 | 0 |

Kite *et al.* (1950)

Table 3.2.
Development of dental caries in rats fed a cariogenic diet and living in either conventional conditions (mixed microbial flora) or under germ-free conditions

| Experiments | Conditions | No. of animals | No. with caries | Mean no. of carious molars |
|---|---|---|---|---|
| Series I | Conventional | 16 | 16 | 4.8 |
| | Germ-free | 13 | 0 | 0 |
| Series II | Conventional | 23 | 23 | 3.2 |
| | Germ-free | 9 | 0 | 0 |

Orland *et al.* (1954).

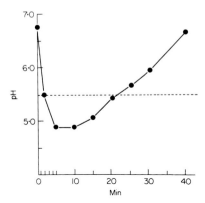

Figure 3.1 Plot of the pH of dental plaque against time: this is commonly known as a Stephan curve. This curve was produced by rinsing with a 10 per cent glucose solution. The broken line represents a typical value of pH below which enamel will dissolve (the 'critical pH').

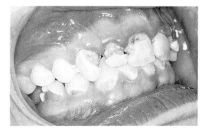

Figure 3.2 Caries initiated at cervical margins and at approximal sites.

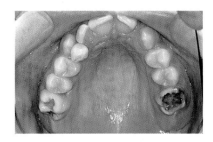

Figure 3.3 Caries originating in pits and fissures of permanent molar teeth.

## Box 3.1  Critical pH

Linked to the Stephan curve is a concept of 'critical pH'. Miller had shown that teeth dissolve in acid, but how acid does it have to be for this to happen in the mouth? The value of pH 5.5 has become accepted as the critical pH below which dental enamel will begin to dissolve because the environment is no longer saturated with enamel mineral. This was first determined by placing enamel in saliva buffered to various pHs, but later (in the 1960s) the value of pH 5.5 was confirmed as being applicable to plaque fluid (extracted by centrifuging plaque). This was important, as caries occurs at the plaque–enamel interface, not at the saliva–enamel interface.

pH of dental plaque was mostly between pH 6.5 and 7.0, but when exposed to sucrose or glucose, the pH of plaque fell rapidly to around pH 5 (Fig. 3.1) within 2–5 min. This rapid fall was then followed by a slow recovery over the next 30–60 min; this plot of plaque pH against time (Fig. 3.1) has become known as the Stephan curve. Work by Geddes and others showed that the predominant acid found in plaque after exposure to sucrose was lactic acid.

The fact that dental caries occurs beneath dental plaque is now quite clear and this distinguishes it from dental erosion which is the dissolution of enamel caused by acids of non-bacterial origin (see Chapter 4). Dental caries occurs in the pits and fissures, approximal surfaces (where teeth abut one another), and around the gingival margin (Figs 3.2 and 3.3). These are areas where plaque accumulates and are quite different from the areas affected by erosion, which are plaque-free exposed surfaces such as the palatal and labial aspects of anterior teeth and the cuspal areas of occlusal surfaces of posterior teeth.

Although both diseases are caused by acids, their aetiology, histopathology, and prevention are quite different. While erosion is surface loss of enamel (as the name implies), the histopathology of dental caries is more complicated, involving sub-surface loss of dental enamel. The reason for this sub-surface dissolution of enamel appears to be related to the diffusion of acids into and mineral out of enamel. The result of these diffusion dynamics is the formation of a relatively well mineralized surface layer of enamel covering the body of the lesion. Eventually, this surface layer gets undermined and weakened so that it collapses

## Box 3.2  Caries or erosion?

| Caries | Erosion |
|---|---|
| Bacterial acids | Extrinsic/intrinsic acids |
| Localized | More widespread |
| Dynamic—demineralization and remineralization | Progressively destructive |
| Rough, chalky areas → cavitation | Concavities with smooth, shiny margins |

and a cavity is formed. Thus, two stages in the caries process can be differentiated—the pre-cavitation stage and the cavity (Figs 3.4 and 3.5). This division is important, as pre-cavitation carious lesions can remineralize or 'heal' while cavities usually have to be filled. A very important part of the preventive care of a patient is to recognize pre-cavitation carious lesions early and to improve the environment to give the enamel the maximum chance to heal.

The ability of early carious lesions (pre-cavitation carious lesions) to remineralize is well understood, but it was not until Backer Dirks presented his observations, over 30 years ago, on the fate of pre-cavitation white spot lesions in the teeth of 8 year old children, that the extent of and potential for remineralization was realized (Table 3.3). Out of 72 lesions, 37 had regressed to become indistinguishable from the surrounding sound enamel during the 7 year observation period.

Dental caries development is clearly, therefore, a dynamic process—the result of an imbalance between demineralization caused by acids formed within plaque which adheres to enamel in areas not adequately cleaned, and remineralization. Removal of plaque is obviously highly desirable, but this is sometimes difficult for all tooth surfaces. Fortunately, plaque removal is not essential as two other factors—saliva and fluoride—play very significant roles in aiding remineralization.

Saliva has many important functions (Table 3.4) but, as far as caries prevention is concerned, buffering and neutralization of plaque acids is a vitally important role. Removal of food from the mouth by physical action is also important. It is these two aspects which bring the pH of dental plaque back to neutrality after its depression following sugar ingestion (Fig. 3.1). Lack of saliva means long and deep Stephan curves, lengthening the time of demineralization and reducing the time when remineralization can occur. The components of saliva most concerned with remineralization are calcium, phosphate, and hydroxyl ions. At neutrality, the concentrations of calcium and phosphate ions in the saliva and plaque fluid are such that the enamel does not dissolve but, as the pH within the plaque falls, plaque fluid is no longer saturated and dissolution occurs. Fortunately, as saliva flow increases, as it does during eating, concentrations of calcium, phosphate and hydroxyl ions increase, aiding remineralization. Thus, increasing salivary flow aids remineralization—a concept which we will return to later in this chapter—and the presence of fluoride enhances this remineralization process.

Thus, it is quite clear that food in the mouth causes dental caries—but what foods? Are there aspects of eating food which influence caries development? And are some foods protective against dental caries?

# Types of study providing evidence for the relationship between diet and caries development

The evidence comes from a number of types of investigation (Box 3.5). Each of these gives useful information but it would be wrong to give equal weight to each type of study. The best evidence comes from studies of the occurrence of dental caries in human populations in relation to their diet. These studies can

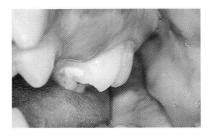

**Figure 3.4** 'White spot' or pre-cavitiation lesion on the mesial surface of the first permanent molar tooth.

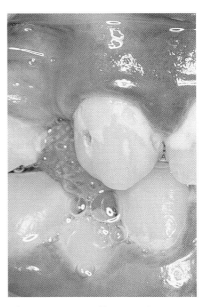

**Figure 3.5.** Maxillary permanent canine tooth showing a variety of carious lesions. Plaque has been removed. Much of the enamel has pre-cavitation carious lesions but cavitation has occurred in several places.

Table 3.3.
The fate of 93 sound surfaces, 72 pre-cavitation lesions, and 19 cavities observed on the buccal surface of maxillary first molars in children aged 8 years, who were subsequently observed until the age of 15 years (7 year observation period)

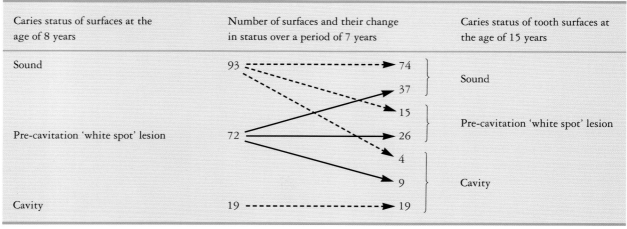

| Caries status of surfaces at the age of 8 years | Number of surfaces and their change in status over a period of 7 years | Caries status of tooth surfaces at the age of 15 years |
|---|---|---|
| Sound | 93 → 74 → 37 | Sound |
| Pre-cavitation 'white spot' lesion | 72 → 15 → 26 → 4 | Pre-cavitation 'white spot' lesion |
| Cavity | 19 → 9 → 19 | Cavity |

Backer Dirks (1966)

Box 3.3 **Key points**

Caries:
 dynamic process
 two stages

Caries development requires:
 presence of plaque
 inadequate mechanical clearance
 low plaque pH
 poor salivary flow

Box 3.4 **Key points**

Components of foods
Patterns of eating
Protective foods

Table 3.4.
The general functions of saliva

| Digestive functions | Protective functions |
|---|---|
| Assisting the mastication of food | Ensuring comfort through lubriction |
| Forming a bolus | Preventing desiccation of oral mucosa, gingivae, and lips |
| Assisting in swallowing of bolus | Antimicrobial |
| Taste perception | lavage |
| Metabolism of starch | bacteriostatic, bactericidal |
| | inhibiting adhesion of bacteria |
| | aggregation of bacteria |
| | Buffering |
| | within saliva |
| | within dental plaque |
| | Removal of toxins (including carcinogens) |
| | Aid speech |

Based on Holt et al. (1988)

either be **observational (epidemiological) studies**, in which the relationships between disease and possible causative and confounding factors are observed, or **interventional studies** in which diets of groups of people are purposefully altered and the effect of this intervention observed. Interventional studies are often known as clinical trials and are rightly taken as the best source of evidence. They are, however, the most difficult to undertake, as large groups of people have to adhere to strict diets for a long enough time for the effect on dental caries increment to be observed. Observational studies are the second best source of evidence and form the largest group. A problem with such studies is that the presence of confounding factors can mask the true effect.

The third source of evidence comes from **animal studies**. Aspects of diet, such as sugar content, frequency of feeding, and content of diet other than sugar can be controlled, and the total experimental period is short. The disadvantages of rodent experiments lie mainly in the difficulties of extrapolating the findings to humans. The fourth method has become known as **enamel slab experiments**. These observe the effects of diet on demineralization in slabs of enamel (cut from extracted teeth) which are held in the mouth of human volunteers in a removable plate constructed like an orthodontic appliance (Fig. 3.6). The fifth type of experiment investigates the effects of foods, meals, or component of foods on the pH of dental plaque. These studies are relatively easy to do, but they measure the 'acidogenicity' of diet rather than 'cariogenicity' and, as such, are only an indication of the possible effect of diet on the development of dental caries. The sixth and final method is the simplest but weakest method: test foods are **incubated** with plaque or saliva (which contains plaque organisms) and the rate of acid production is recorded. In some experiments, whole enamel, powdered enamel, or calcium phosphate are added to the saliva/substrate mixture and the rate of dissolution of mineral is taken as a measure of cariogenic potential.

Evidence from all these sources will be used to indicate relevant aspects of cariogenicity of foods and the strengths and drawbacks of each type of evidence needs to borne in mind.

---

**Box 3.5 Types of study**

1. Observational (epidemiological) studies
2. Interventional studies
3. Animal studies
4. Enamel slab experiments
5. Acidogenicity studies
6. Incubation studies

---

**Box 3.6 Confounding factors in epidemiology**

The most common concern over confounding is that it may create the appearance of a cause–effect relationship where, in reality, one doesn't exist. Confounding occurs when the effects of two 'exposures' or 'risk factors' have not been separated, and it is incorrectly concluded that the effect is due to one rather than the other variable. If possible 'confounders' can be identified and measured, modern statistical techniques can remove their effect.

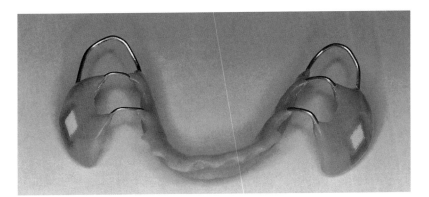

**Figure 3.6** An example of an acrylic resin appliance showing two buccal flanges each containing a terylene mesh-covered slab of enamel. Reproduced with permission of *New Zealand Dental Journal*

# Components of foods

Foods consist, broadly, of carbohydrates, fats, proteins, minerals, and vitamins. As mentioned earlier, Miller showed over 100 years ago that carbohydrates incubated with saliva produced acid—thus, it is reasonable to give close attention to the cariogenicity of carbohydrates. But carbohydrates themselves vary considerably—from simple mono- and disaccharide sugars, to short-chain oligosaccharides, to complex carbohydrates (polysaccharides). Polysaccharides are either starches, which are metabolized, or non-starch polysaccharides (NSP) commonly known as 'fibre' and are mostly not metabolized. Another class of carbohydrate derivatives of special interest to us are the polyols.

Since people eat foods and advice is usually given in terms of foods, we will consider types of foods such as milk, fruit, vegetables, as well as the components of foods.

Fats and proteins will require little attention as they are non-cariogenic. Fats have been considered to be marginally anti-cariogenic by aiding clearance of food from the mouth, so making carbohydrate less available to plaque organisms. Minerals relevant to caries prevention are calcium, phosphorus, and fluoride, while vitamins are not generally considered to have a direct role in caries prevention. Vitamin D has received some attention because of its role in calcification (see Chapter 2) and its importance in caries aetiology is still unclear, especially as there is some patchy evidence that it may have a post-eruptive (intraoral) caries preventive effect. Attention will therefore be given to the carbohydrates and possible protective factors in foods.

# Sugars and caries

Because sugars are metabolized so easily by plaque bacteria into acids, much attention has been devoted to clarifying their undoubted role in caries development. In fact, well over 1000 articles have been published on this topic covering all types of investigations. Only the most important aspects will be considered here, to enable conclusions to be drawn and reasons for advice appreciated.

## Types of sugar

Relevant dietary sugars are sucrose, glucose, fructose, maltose, lactose, and galactose. The sugar most commonly associated with dental caries is sucrose and indeed sucrose has been labelled 'the arch criminal of dental caries'. This view was based first on the results of animal experiments, which often demonstrated high caries scores in groups receiving diets containing sucrose compared with other sugars and, second, sucrose is unique in its ability to encourage extensive dextran production in plaque. In recent years, the role of dextran in the development of dental caries has been considered to be less important. The Turku sugar studies showed little difference in caries development between sucrose and fructose groups and enamel slab experiments have supported the view that sucrose, fructose, and maltose have rather similar cariogenic potential. These sugars also produce similar Stephan curves. The ability of sucrose to produce more caries than other sugars in animals is now recognized to be due, largely, to the common practice of super-infecting the mouths of rats with specific organisms in order to standardize this variable between groups of animals. These organisms happen to be those that are particularly good at metabolizing sucrose, thus leading to the result of higher caries scores in the animals receiving the sucrose diet. Nevertheless, no sugar has been shown to be more cariogenic than sucrose and, since it is the most widely available dietary sugar, it is not surprising that it has been subject of the greatest criticism. There seems to be little difference in the cariogenicity of glucose, fructose, and maltose, if evidence from animal, enamel slab, plaque pH, and incubation experiments are considered, but the same sources of evidence show that lactose is less cariogenic. What little data there are on galactose indicate a cariogenicity similar to that of lactose.

## Sugars in society

Sugar consumption really took off with the commercial mass production of sugar cane and refining of sugar cane some 150 years ago. Most of the cane was grown and harvested in warmer climates but refining was in the hands of European companies. Much later, sugar beet was grown in temperate climates and has superseded cane sugar to some extent. Recent advances in enzyme technology have enabled a wide variety of sweeteners—commonly glucose syrup or, especially in the USA, fructose syrup—to be produced from a variety of starchy foods such as corn, other grains, and potatoes. Sweet foods such as honey have always been available, but usually as a luxury: now the tables are turned and sugar is one of the cheapest of foods. Consumption of sugar increased first in developed countries and with it came a wave of dental caries. Figures 3.7 and 3.8 illustrate this for the UK. Caries data for Fig. 3.7 came from archaeological material.

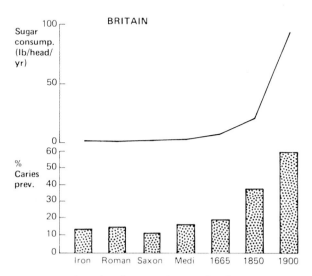

**Figure 3.7** Percentage dental caries prevalence related to mean sugar consumption in British populations from the Iron Age to modern times. Source: Moore & Corbett (1978)

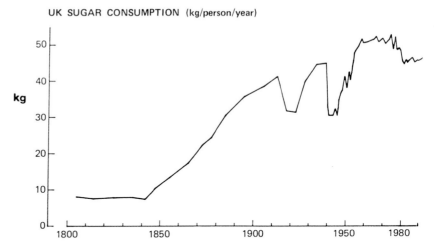

UK SUGAR CONSUMPTION (kg/person/year)

**Figure 3.8** UK sugar consumption over the last 200 years.

Epidemiological surveys during the past 100 years have shown dental caries to be a significant public health problem since 1900, dipping during the two World Wars, before reaching its highest level in the 1950s and 1960s, in parallel with sugar consumption. Caries experience has declined rapidly since the 1970s, almost certainly due to the widespread use of fluoride. Sugar consumption has been low in the developing world but, with increasing wealth and trade, sugar consumption is increasing in the Middle East, south and south-east Asia, and in central and south America. It is in these areas that the highest levels of dental caries are now found in young children. There are several well documented examples of dental caries experience being recorded before and after a change in a country from a low to a high sugar diet. In each case, caries increased in parallel with the change in diet.

There have been several attempts to correlate sugar consumption in countries with their caries experience. This is of necessity fairly crude epidemiology, as sugar consumption data are of variable accuracy and apply to all ages, while caries data are often based on small surveys and are usually age specific (data for 12 year olds are often used). Nevertheless, these tend to show a positive correlation between sugar consumption and caries experience, although this is more obvious in developing countries and less obvious in developed countries where the effect of fluoride-based preventive programmes has an important influence (Fig. 3.9).

There has been a marked decline in caries experience in children in several European countries over the past 25 years. By far the most important reason for this is, almost certainly, the widespread use of fluorides, especially in toothpastes. However, it is worth making some remarks about diet. First, the way sugar is consumed has changed: sugar confectionery has given way to chocolate confectionery, which may be less cariogenic (see later). Second, non-sugar sweeteners have made substantial inroads into the confectionery market (see later), which may explain part of the decline in caries in countries such as Switzerland and

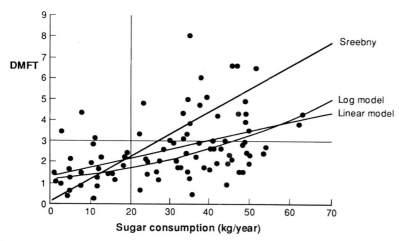

**Figure 3.9** Number of decayed, missing, or filled teeth (DMFT) against estimated sugar consumption for 90 countries. The best-fitting regression model, the log model, is shown together with the linear model. Also shown is the linear model found by Sreebny using an earlier data set. Reproduced with permission of *British Dental Journal*.

Finland. Third, in the USA, high fructose corn syrup (HFCS) has displaced sucrose as the major sweetener in manufactured products and some people believe that this sweetener is less cariogenic than sucrose. Nevertheless, in simple terms it is reasonable to conclude that the rise in caries prevalence and severity in the world has been due to the rise in availability and consumption of sugars, while the caries decline has been due to the use of fluorides. The interplay between the opposing effects of sugar and fluoride is a very important topic, especially from the public health perspective, and will be returned to later in Chapter 9.

Sources of sugars in the diets of adolescents in the UK are given in Table 3.5. Confectionery is the largest source followed by soft drinks and table sugar. Because confectionery and soft drinks are major sources of sugars, their effects on teeth have been investigated extensively. Designs of epidemiological surveys have varied much, with some examining young children, some older children, and some adults. On the whole, these studies show positive correlations between confectionery and caries, especially in young children. One of the drawbacks of the commonly used cross-sectional design of study is that it compares lifetime experience of dental caries with a once-only assessment of diet, with the assumption that diets have not changed over several years previously. While this may be true for young children, it is less tenable in older children and adults. A better design is the longitudinal design, where diet and caries development are measured over the same time period. There have been only a few of these, but their results again indicate the importance of the consumption of dietary sugars, especially confectionery. There have been far fewer studies specifying soft drinks as a risk factor in dental caries. It is not clear why this is—it could be that sugars in solution (usually about 10 per cent) are less damaging than sugars in solids and more retentive forms.

Box 3.7

A *cross-sectional* epidemiological study examines the population just once: for example, a survey of dental caries in 12 year old children. Cross-sectional studies can be repeated, to investigate change in disease over time, but the same subjects are not re-examined.

In a *longitudinal* study, the subjects are re-examined after a stated period (for example, 2 years) to measure change in disease in those people.

Table 3.5.
Mean daily intake of non-milk extrinsic sugars, milk and intrinsic sugars, and total sugars from various dietary sources (in grams and as a percentage of sugars intake) by UK adolescents

| | Non-milk extrinsic | | Intrinsic and milk | | Total | |
|---|---|---|---|---|---|---|
| | g | % | g | % | g | % |
| Confectionery | 30 | 33 | 1 | 4 | 31 | 26 |
| Soft drinks | 24 | 27 | 0 | 0 | 24 | 20 |
| Biscuits and cakes | 10 | 11 | 1 | 3 | 11 | 9 |
| Table sugar | 11 | 12 | 0 | 0 | 11 | 9 |
| Milk | 0 | 0 | 10 | 35 | 10 | 8 |
| Sweet puddings | 5 | 6 | 3 | 12 | 9 | 7 |
| Breakfast cereals | 5 | 5 | 0 | 1 | 5 | 4 |
| Fruit | 0 | 0 | 5 | 17 | 5 | 4 |
| Syrups and preserves | 2 | 2 | 1 | 3 | 3 | 3 |
| Other sources | 3 | 4 | 7 | 24 | 10 | 9 |
| All sources | 90 | 100 | 28 | 100 | 118 | 100 |

Rugg-Gunn *et al.* (1993)

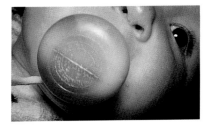

**Figure 3.10** A reservoir feeder containing sweetened fruit juice being used by a baby.

Moving to a younger age group, there is no doubt that fruit-flavoured infant drinks are major causes of caries in infants and young children. These drinks are commonly given to the infant in bottles or reservoir (dinky) feeders and used as a pacifier (Figs 3.10 and 3.11). Several reviews of these surveys have been published—the most comprehensive by Winter in 1980. Winter, Holt, and colleagues have undertaken studies of this problem in pre-school children in Camden, London (Table 3.6). As can be seen, around 10 per cent of children

Table 3.6.
The prevalence of dental caries and the prevalence of 'rampant caries' (caries involving deciduous incisor teeth) in pre-school London children, 1993–4

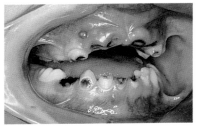

**Figure 3.11** An intraoral view of the baby in Figure 3.10 showing the caries attack and anterior open bite, as a consequence of the feeder habit.

| Age (months) | *n* | Dental caries prevalence (%) | Prevalence of rampant caries (%) |
|---|---|---|---|
| 12–23 | 198 | 6 | 2 |
| 24–35 | 150 | 11 | 6 |
| 36–47 | 132 | 29 | 14 |
| 48–59 | 85 | 34 | 13 |

Holt *et al.* (1996)

Table 3.7.
The number of decayed, missing, or filled primary teeth (dmft) in children aged 9 months to 6 years who had been taking sugar-containing liquid oral medicines frequently, long term, compared with a matched control group

| Group | Number | Mean dmft |
|-------|--------|-----------|
| Medicine | 44 | 5.6 |
| Control | 47 | 1.3 |

Roberts & Roberts (1979)

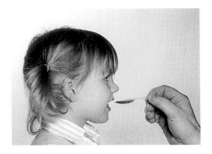

**Figure 3.12** Many liquid oral medicines are heavily sweetened to increase palatability and thus compliance.

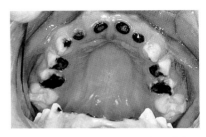

**Figure 3.13** Extensive caries of the primary dentition of this 7 year old child who required frequent courses of sweetened liquid oral medicines as a toddler.

have extensive dental caries (often known as rampant caries) and in many cases this was related to the use of bottles or comforters containing sugared fruit-flavoured drinks.

Medicines for children are often given as a liquid orally (Fig. 3.12). Most of these contain sugar, often up to 70 per cent concentration, to make them more palatable. For many children, the course of medicine is brief and the added sugar burden negligible. But there is a significant group of children who require medicines daily, for various conditions from epilepsy to chronic infections (Fig. 3.13). These children are at significant risk of dental caries, as can be seen in Table 3.7. Medicines sometimes have to be given just before or during sleep, a time when salivary flow is low, increasing the risk of caries. These children are already ill and it is highly undesirable to give the child the further burden of dental caries.

## Frequency of intake of sugars and caries development

There is much evidence that the frequency of intake of sugars has a considerable influence on dental caries development. The pH of dental plaque falls rapidly when sugars are eaten (Fig. 3.1). There is some disagreement as to the length of the recovery period but, regardless of this, it is logical to conclude that the more occasions sugar is taken, the greater the number of times plaque pH will fall below a level where demineralization can occur (the critical pH). The converse is—the longer the time plaque pH is at a low level, the less time there is for remineralization to occur.

The second indicator of the importance of frequency is animal experiments. The studies of König and colleagues in 1968 showed clearly that dental caries experience increased with increasing frequency of intake of sugar, even when the total amount of sugar eaten by all groups of rats per day was the same (Table 3.8).

Third, the patients in a study in the Vipeholm Hospital in Sweden who ate sugary foods between meals as well as at meals developed much more caries than patients who were fed sugar only at meals. The groups which consumed the most sweets between meals (the 24 toffees per day groups) developed the most caries.

Table 3.8.

The mean dental caries severity and daily food intake in five groups of rats fed at different frequencies per day; six animals per group

| Group | Eating frequency per day | No of fissure lesions | Daily food intake (g) |
|-------|--------------------------|-----------------------|------------------------|
| 1 | 12 | 0.7 | 6.0 |
| 2 | 18 | 2.2 | 6.0 |
| 3 | 24 | 4.0 | 6.0 |
| 4 | 30 | 4.7 | 6.0 |
| 5 | *ad lib* | 4.2 | 11.7 |

König *et al.* (1968)

However, there is also evidence that the amount of sugar consumed is an important factor as well. Animal experiments have been conducted on the effect of altering the concentration of sugars in the diet fed to rats and, since the frequency of feeding was similar in all groups, as the concentrations of sugars increased so did the total amount of sugar in the diet (Fig. 3.14). As can be seen, caries increased with increasing concentration and amount of sugars in the diet.

In most of the extensive list of epidemiological studies referred to earlier in this chapter, the weight of sugars consumed rather than frequency of consumption was measured and related to the development of dental caries. For example, in the worldwide comparisons, sugar supply was measured in grams per person

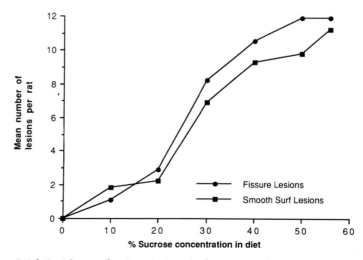

**Figure 3.14** Incidence of carious lesions in fissures (circles) and smooth surfaces (squares) in rats fed diets containing 0, 10, 20, 30, 40, 51, and 56 per cent sucrose. Reproduced with permission of *Caries Research*.

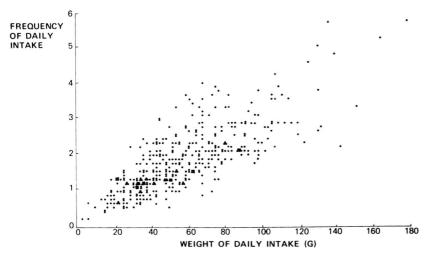

**Figure 3.15** Plot of the frequency of intake per day against the weight consumed per day, of confectionery, by 12–14 year old children in north-east England. The correlation coefficient is high at +0.77.

per day. It was also noted that dental caries experience increased as sugar consumption increased, and decreased as the amount of sugar consumed decreased. It is very likely that frequency of eating sugar rose as the amount of sugar available rose and, in free living people (as opposed to laboratory animals), a high positive correlation between amount and frequency of eating sugary foods can be safely assumed: data supporting this are given in Fig. 3.15. Thus, it is sensible to advise cutting down on both frequency of consumption of sugar as well as the total amount of sugar consumed.

## Fruit, vegetables, and dental caries

For years, fresh fruit and vegetables have been regarded as being good for dental health and often used as a symbol in dental health campaigns. This was partly because they were seen as a 'mouth cleanser'—nature's toothbrush. Philip of Macedon believed that every meal should be followed by the acid of fruit in order to cleanse the mouth and aid digestion. Consequently, he made a ruling throughout his household that every meal must terminate with the eating of an apple.

Several studies have shown that apples do not remove plaque or improve gingival health, and so this aspect of tooth cleaning can be dismissed. However, it is possible that the stimulation of salivary flow by eating firm fresh fruit or vegetables (such as apples or carrots) could help prevent dental caries. This has been put to the test in four studies, two in the UK and two in the USA. None of these studies were perfectly conducted—in two no effect was observed of eating apples after the last meal of the day or eating pieces of raw carrot after midday meal in school. In the other two studies, there was a hint (which reached statistical significance in one study) of less caries development in subjects who consumed apples (or pieces of apples for children) at the end of each meal.

Other studies have looked at the cariogenicity of fresh fruit as part of the general diet. Very few studies have investigated vegetables and their cariogenicity has never been considered an issue. Many studies have reported lower caries experience in people with higher fruit intake while other studies have shown no effect. Caries development has been measured in children and adults consuming lacto-vegetarian diets—the results are mixed, with a study of children in Australia reporting very low caries experience, while a study of adults in Finland reported no effect. Only in one study has fruit eating been associated with higher caries experience (Table 3.9). The subjects were random samples of adults of both sexes aged 15 years or more who lived on farms in three districts of south-western Cape Province in South Africa, for a minimum of 8 years. These three districts grew predominantly apple, grape, or grain crops; the grain district served as a control area. Dental caries was significantly higher in adults from the apple growing area than from the grape growing area, and the dental caries experience of both these groups was significantly higher than that observed in the control area. One unexplained feature of these results can be seen in the two right-hand columns of Table 3.9 in that all the difference between groups was due to missing teeth (MT) and the number of decayed and filled teeth (DFT) did not differ between groups.

The question of dried fruit is a difficult one. Aristotle is quoted as saying that 'dried figs produce damage to the teeth'. Consumption of dried fruits is not great and there have been no epidemiological studies or clinical trials to investigate their cariogenicity. There have, though, been extensive animal studies which have shown that dried figs, dates, and raisins cause caries in rats. Such studies, though, are difficult to extrapolate to people as, in rat-feeding experiments, these foods have to be dried and ground finely to enable the rats to eat them, and this may encourage the impaction of these powdered foods in fissures, increasing caries development.

The last form in which fruits are consumed is juices. In contrast to the above rather equivocal evidence regarding whole fruit and dental caries, there is much evidence to incriminate the frequent and prolonged use of sugared fruit drinks and fruit-flavoured drinks as an important cause of dental caries in young children (Table 3.10).

Table 3.9.
Effect of high consumption of apples or grapes on experience of dental caries in South African adults

| Farm workers | $n$ | DMFT* | MT | DFT |
|---|---|---|---|---|
| Apple growers | 95 | 24 | 20 | 4 |
| Grape growers | 109 | 17 | 13 | 4 |
| Grain growers | 50 | 10 | 4 | 6 |

* Differences between groups were all significant ($p < 0.05$).
MT: mean number of decayed or filled teeth per person.
DFT: mean number of decayed or filled teeth per person.
Grobler & Blignaut (1989)

Table 3.10.
Proportion of pre-school children with any decay
experience according to reported drinking practices at night

| | 2.5–3.5 years | 3.5–4.5 years |
|---|---|---|
| Type of drink in bed | | |
| Drink + non-milk extrinsic sugars | 40 | 35 |
| Milk | 15 | 19 |
| | | |
| Container usually used | | |
| Bottle | 21 | 42 |
| Feeder cup | 18 | 18 |
| Mug/cup/glass | 10 | 28 |

Department of Health (1995) NDNS

Box 3.8 **Classification of sugars**

*Intrinsic sugars* are sugars present in whole fruit and vegetables.

*Milk sugars* are sugars (lactose and galactose) present in milk.

*Non-milk extrinsic sugars* are, as the name implies, all the other sugars in the diet. These sugars are added to provide sweetness and constitute some 60–70 per cent of total dietary sugars.

## Summary regarding fruit and vegetables

- Fresh fruit, dried fruit, and fruit juices are capable of causing dental caries but their role as a cause of dental caries in humans differs, as indicated below.

- Sugared fruit-flavoured drinks, when used in a comforter bottle, are a significant cause of dental caries in young children. Virtually all reports mention fruit-flavoured drinks and not pure fruit juices as a cause of dental caries. However, this may be due to the greater availability in the past of sugared fruit-flavoured drinks compared with pure fruit juices.

- As eaten by humans, fresh fruits appear to be of low cariogenicity. Citrus fruits have not been associated with the development of dental caries. Large consumption of apples and grapes has been associated with high caries prevalence, but this has only been recorded in one study.

- Consumption of dried fruit is low and it is not possible to give advice confidently on their cariogenicity. It is possible that dried fruit causes caries but this does not appear to be a significant problem.

# Milk and dental caries

Milk is one of the main sources of sugar in the human diet. For infants, it is the only source and its importance declines after weaning, so by early adolescence the 12 g of lactose consumed per child per day contributes about 10 per cent of total intake of sugars. Cow's milk soon supersedes human milk as the type of milk consumed in most countries.

Various components of milk have been considered to be protective against dental caries, namely the minerals, casein, and other lipid and protein components. Cheese, a product of milk, has been the subject of much interest among dental scientists over the past three decades, and is considered by many to have substantial protective properties against caries. The evidence for these claims of a protective action of milk and milk-based products will be considered later.

Both human milk and cow's milk contain lactose, about 7 g/100 g in human and about 5 g/100 g in cow's milk (Table 3.11). These amounts could be sufficient to classify milks as cariogenic, but it should be remembered that lactose is the least cariogenic of the common dietary sugars. In addition, the high concentrations of calcium and phosphorus in milks will help to prevent dissolution of enamel (which is largely calcium and phosphate) and other factors may be protective as well. The amounts of calcium and phosphorus in human and cow's milk are quite different, thus these two milks may have rather different cariogenic potentials.

There have been a few reports of dental caries being associated with on-demand breastfeeding and, more rarely, prolonged bottle-feeding with cow's milk or formula feed (Fig. 3.16). However, these cases are fairly exceptional, as feeding was on-demand and prolonged over several years. Further aspects of breastfeeding and bottle-feeding will be discussed in Chapter 7.

Epidemiological studies, on the whole, have associated breastfeeding with low dental caries experience. To what extent this is a direct relationship or secondary to economic status, which is linked to both breastfeeding and, inversely, to consumption of sucrose-containing foods, is unclear.

Evidence from animal experiments not only indicates that cow's milk is non-cariogenic but also strongly suggests an anti-cariogenic effect. The extensive studies of Stephan labelled milk as non-cariogenic. Supplementation of a cariogenic diet with cow's milk substantially reduced dental caries incidence and this was not due to a reduced consumption of the cariogenic diet. A severe test of the cariogenic or cariostatic properties of milk was carried out by Bowen and colleagues using desalivated rats, which are therefore much more susceptible to caries. Rats given milk or lactose-reduced milk remained essentially caries-free, while those given the same amount of sucrose or lactose in water developed caries.

Thus, in conclusion, for practical purposes milk can be considered non-cariogenic. Indeed, cow's milk may be a non-cariogenic drink suitable for use as

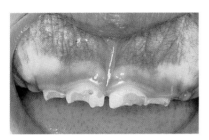

**Figure 3.16** Typical caries distribution on maxillary primary incisor teeth in a child who has been breastfed, on demand, especially overnight, for more than 16 months.

Table 3.11.

The average lactose, calcium, and phosphorus content of human and bovine (cow's) milk

|  | Lactose (g/100 ml) | Calcium (mg/100 ml) | Phosphorus (mg/100 ml) |
|---|---|---|---|
| Human milk | 7.0 | 33 | 15 |
| Bovine milk | 4.8 | 125 | 96 |

Darke (1976)

an artificial saliva in caries-prone xerostomic patients, since it appears to have caries-protective properties. Human milk is likely to have greater cariogenic potential but dental caries in human infants due to breastfeeding is very rare and usually associated with prolonged, on-demand feeding.

# Starches and dental caries

'It's not just the sugar in foods and drinks that causes acid attacks. We now know that all foods which contain carbohydrate—either sugars or cooked starch—can do the same'.

This statement by a confectionery manufacturer is true if only the weakest form of evidence—incubation studies—is considered. To recall Miller's studies of 110 years ago, when carbohydrate foods (such as bread) were incubated with saliva, acid was produced and the acidic incubate was capable of demineralizing tooth enamel. Saliva contains the enzyme amylase which breaks down starch molecules, and bacteria, which then metabolize the short-chain saccharides to acids. This type of incubation experiment has been repeated very many times. Overall, these experiments do not provide very much useful information concerning the cariogenicity of starchy foods, other than showing that acids can be produced from starchy foods.

What of the other sources of evidence? We will work our way from the weakest (incubation experiments) to the strongest (human studies) forms of evidence. First, plaque pH experiments. It is important to realize that these investigate acidogenicity not cariogenicity and any 'protective factors' present in starchy foods would not affect the measurement of acidogenicity, but would decrease cariogenicity since they affect solubility not acid production. Almost all of the plaque pH experiments investigating starch have been carried out either using the sampling method or the indwelling glass electrode method of measuring plaque pH. The sampling method has tended to indicate that cooked starch, or starchy foods, are less acidogenic than sugar or high sugar foods and that uncooked starches are virtually non-acidogenic. Conversely, indwelling glass electrode experiments have shown that starch is capable of depressing plaque pH below what is commonly called the critical pH (pH 5.5). Whether this accurately reflects what occurs naturally in humans is open to question, since indwelling glass electrodes tend to give an all-or-nothing response to foods—any carbohydrate-containing food leading to a maximum drop in pH. This feature makes the application of the method to evaluating relative cariogenicity of snack foods difficult, as foods such as bread, judged to be of low cariogenicity by other methods, appeared highly cariogenic and the technique has mainly found favour in verifying the low acidogenicity of sugar substitutes.

Enamel slab experiments are a little nearer reality since demineralization and remineralization usually occur *in vivo*. Experiments which have investigated the cariogenicity of starch have indicated that cooked starch is about one quarter as cariogenic as sucrose.

A large number of animal experiments have been undertaken with rather variable results. Raw starches appear to have very low cariogenicity while cooked starches cause dental caries, but the amount is less than that caused by sucrose.

Mixtures of starch and sucrose cause more dental caries than starch alone and the amount of dental caries was positively related to the amount of sugar in the mixture. The degree of processing of starch in manufactured foods influences the development of dental caries in rats, due to the partial hydrolysis of starch (for example in fried potato chips and extruded starchy snack foods). Clearly, animal experiments are useful in giving some indication of the cariogenicity of foods in humans, but caution in their interpretation is necessary.

Human observational and interventional studies are the only types of study which actually record the development of caries in people and as such should provide the most valid estimate of cariogenicity. For many thousands of years, starchy foods have formed the staple diet of humans with very little caries development. Even now, in countries consuming high starch, low sugar diets, caries remains low. It appears that only when sugar consumption increases does caries increase. Of course, starchy foods have become more processed—flour is heat treated and finely ground, which breaks down the starch granules and some of the long-chain starch molecules—which may make them more cariogenic. Frequency of eating may have increased also (although there is no evidence for this), but it is unlikely that these aspects explain the great rise in caries which has occurred in developed countries—the rise in consumption of sugars remains by far the most reasonable explanation.

On a worldwide basis, it is interesting to look at correlations between dental caries experience, sugar consumption, and starch consumption: this has been done using information from 47 countries. Partial correlation analyses were made first between caries experience and cereal availability, controlling for sugar availability. The results of these analyses showed that correlations between caries and cereal were reduced to near zero when sugar was controlled for, indicating that cereal availability did not affect caries experience. On the other hand, the strong positive relation between caries experience and sugar availability was unaffected by standardizing the data on cereal availability, thus indicating that sugar availability had a real effect on caries experience.

There have been a number of reports of people living in modern western societies who habitually eat very low amounts of sugar, either because they possess inborn errors of metabolism or for other reasons. They consume high starch diets. Hereditary fructose intolerance (HFI) is a rare inherited disorder of fructose metabolism in which illness is caused by an intake of fructose (and sucrose which contains fructose). The diets and dental caries status of 17 HFI subjects have been compared with those of 14 control subjects who were unaffected and mostly blood relatives. The mean ages were 29 years for the HFI subjects and 27 years for the control subjects. The respective mean DMFT scores were 2.1 and 14.3, while the mean daily sucrose consumption was 3 g and 48 g, and the respective mean daily starch consumption was 160 g and 140 g. The finding that the HFI subjects consumed high levels of starch (higher than the control subjects) and yet developed minimal levels of dental caries must indicate that starch is not particularly caries inducive.

There is information on the dental health of children brought up in communities in which sugar intake has been restricted. Dietary starch would have come principally from potatoes, rice, and wholemeal flour. Caries experience was very low in these children compared with Australian children living outside the home.

Evidence from cross-sectional and longitudinal observation studies tends to show that dietary sugars are positively associated with the development of dental caries, while dietary starches are not. In some of these studies the effects of possible confounding factors such as fluoride and tooth-brushing have been removed and the results were unchanged.

One relevant interventional study is the Turku study, which will be discussed later as it was a major trial of substitution of dietary sugars by a non-sugar sweetener. This trial of substitution of sucrose by xylitol resulted in a substantial reduction in the incidence of dental caries. Since starch intake was unaltered, dietary starch cannot have contributed significantly to the development of dental caries in these human subjects.

## Summary regarding starchy foods

- Cooked staple starchy foods, such as rice, potatoes, spaghetti, and bread are of low cariogenicity in humans.
- Finely ground and heat-treated starch can cause dental caries, but less so than that caused by sugars.
- The addition of sugar increases the cariogenicity of cooked starchy foods.
- Less refined starchy foods may have properties which help to protect teeth from dental caries. These properties, which will be discussed later, include
  - (a) a fibre content such that the food has to be chewed vigorously, which aids removal of food from the mouth and increases salivary flow; and
  - (b) possible protective factors which may protect the teeth from dissolution.

# Oligosaccharides

Advances in food technology have encouraged the development of medium-chain glucose polymers—these can be called by the broad term 'oligosaccharides'. Food manufacturers will use those that have the most appropriate properties for any particular food product—for example, some are sweet-tasting and some are not. They are usually made by enzymatic breakdown of starchy foods, such as corn, other grains, and potatoes. When a polymer has a dextrose equivalent of less than 20 it is called a maltodextrin. Very often products such as corn-starch syrups have a mixture of mono, di, tri, tetra, penta, hexa, and heptasaccharides, together with 13–45 per cent of saccharides with chain length greater than 7. The monosaccharides, disaccharides, and trisaccharides can be metabolized readily by the plaque organism *Streptococcus mutans*.

The amount of information available on the effect of these oligosaccharides on dental health is limited, both in number of studies and in scope. Results from plaque pH studies and rat experiments suggest that their cariogenicity is between those of starch and sugars. This seems logical as the longer and more complicated the glucose polymer chain, the longer it would take to be divided by saliva and plaque enzymes, and metabolized to acids by plaque bacteria.

| Bulk sweeteners | Intense sweeteners |
| --- | --- |
| Sorbitol | Saccharin |
| Mannitol | Acesulfame K[a] |
| Hydrogenated | Aspartame[a] |
| glucose syrup[a] | Thaumatin[a] |
| Isomalt[a] | |
| Xylitol[a] | |
| Lactitol[b] | |
| Maltitol[c] | |

[a] Permitted 1982.
[b] Permitted 1988.
[c] Permitted 1996.

Box 3.9

Are non-sugar sweeteners
non-cariogenic?

Can plaque flora adapt to
metabolize these non-sugar
sweeteners?

Do any of these sweeteners have a
positive anti-caries effect?

Are there any undesirable
side-effects of using non-sugar
sweeteners?

What is the likely gain from
sugar substitution?

# Non-sugar sweeteners

Because of the predominant role of sugars as a cause of dental caries, and because the sweet taste of sugars is popular, it is not surprising that the use of non-sugar sweeteners in place of cariogenic sweeteners has been investigated enthusiastically. Their most important role, so far, has been in the manufacture of sugar-free confectionery and chewing gums. This is sensible, as confectionery is easily the biggest source of dietary sugars; confectionery is made and marketed for frequent eating, making it doubly dangerous if it contains sugar. Other important roles for non-sugar sweeteners are in soft drinks, table-top sweeteners (for tea or coffee), and in liquid oral medicines.

A very large number of sweet compounds are known, but relatively few are permitted to be used in foods and those that are varies from country to country. Those that are permitted at present in the UK are listed in Table 3.12. Seventeen years ago, only two bulk sweeteners and one intense sweetener were allowed: the expansion since then indicates a growing interest in non-sugar sweeteners. Manufacturers of non-sugar sweeteners are keen to develop new products with improved properties, and many of these have been approved by government food safety authorities. Food manufacturers have been able to use them to improve their products and the public have wished to buy these products. It would be unwise to expect rapid changes in the use of sweeteners although this has happened in some products, such as chewing gums which are now largely sugar-free.

It is convenient to divide non-sugar sweeteners into bulk sweeteners and intense sweeteners (Table 3.13). Bulk sweeteners are approximately the same sweetness as sucrose, gram for gram; they also provide calories, almost as much as sucrose. Many of the bulk sweeteners are sugar alcohols or 'polyols'. Intense sweeteners provide very little or, more usually, no energy and are very many times as sweet as sucrose.

## Sorbitol

Sorbitol is used extensively as a non-sugar sweetener in confectionery, chewing gum, liquid oral medicines, and toothpastes. It used to be used in diabetic foods, but these are less important in modern treatment of diabetes. The negative heat of dissolution is used advantageously in mints, which have a pleasant cool taste.

The cariogenicity of sorbitol has been tested extensively in several types of study. Sorbitol is fermented slowly by plaque organisms, but the rate is very much slower than that for glucose and sucrose. Plaque pH and enamel slab experiments have all testified to the low acidogenicity and cariogenicity of sorbitol. Almost all of the clinical trials of sorbitol on dental health in humans have tested sorbitol in chewing gum; one trial of sorbitol sweets gave positive results. The results of clinical trials of sorbitol-containing chewing gum will be considered later—briefly these trials showed sorbitol-containing gum to be non-cariogenic.

Concern has been expressed that oral flora may adapt to sorbitol so that it loses its safe-for-teeth property; the subject has been reviewed extensively and in the light of current evidence, frequent or long-term use of sorbitol is unlikely to represent any increased risk of dental caries in normal people.

Table 3.13.
Bulk and intense sweeteners

| Agent | Sweetness (cf. sucrose) | Cariogenicity | Clinical trials | Uses | Special effects | Calories |
|---|---|---|---|---|---|---|
| **Bulk sweeteners** | | | | | | |
| Sorbitol | 0.5 | Virtually non-cariogenic (substantial evidence) | Yes—gums and sweets | Confectionery; medicines; gum; toothpaste | Negative heat of dissolution | Yes |
| Mannitol | 0.7 | Virtually non-cariogenic (some evidence) | One | Dusting powder on chewing gum | Negative heat of dissolution + non-hygroscopic | Yes |
| Maltitol | 0.7 | Virtually non-cariogenic (some evidence) | None | Gums | – | Yes |
| Lactitol | 0.3 | Virtually non-cariogenic (some evidence) | None | Confectionery | – | Yes |
| Xylitol | 1.0 | Non-cariogenic; anti-cariogenic? | Yes—in foods and in gums | Confectionery, gums, toothpaste | Negative heat of dissolution | Yes |
| Lycasin (hydrogenated glucose syrup) | 0.7 | Between sorbitol and xylitol (substantial evidence) | None | Confectionery; chewing gum; medicines | – | Yes |
| Isomalt | 0.5 | Virtually non-cariogenic (substantial evidence) | None | Chocolate | – | Yes |
| **Intense sweeteners** | | | | | | |
| Saccharin | 500 | ? Inhibits caries | None | Table top; low calorie foods + drinks | Bitter taste | No |
| Acesulfame potassium | 130 | No effect | None | Low energy drinks; confectionery; foods; preserves | – | No |
| Aspartame | 200 | No effect | None | Soft drinks; dried/frozen foods; gums | To be avoided in people with PKU | Very few |
| Thaumatin | 3000 | No effect | None | Flavour enhancer in pharmaceuticals with other sweeteners; in soft drinks | Liquorice after-taste | No |

## Mannitol

Mannitol is a non-sugar sweetener used in confectionery and chewing gum (especially as a dusting powder as it is non-hygroscopic), but it is less popular than sorbitol, partly because of its higher price. There is much less information on the dental effects of mannitol compared with sorbitol. When mannitol and sorbitol were tested in the same experiments, they had similar dental properties. There have been no clinical trials where mannitol has been the sole sweetener.

## Xylitol

Xylitol has been subject to all types of study. In all of these, it appears to be non-cariogenic. Of more interest is whether it has a specific anti-caries action—a positive effect rather than a neutral effect. This will be discussed later in a section on chewing gums.

Microbiological studies have shown clearly that xylitol is not metabolized by most of the organisms in plaque. A few strains are able to degrade xylitol to acids, but the rate is very slow and these organisms occur in plaque in insignificant numbers. Even after 2 years use, plaque organisms did not adapt to metabolize xylitol. Plaque pH, animal, and enamel slab experiments have all indicated the non-acidogenicity and non-cariogenicity of xylitol.

The Turku sugar studies were one of the milestones in dental caries research. The main study tested the effects on development of dental caries over 2 years, in adults, of almost total substitution of normal dietary sugars with xylitol. This was a great organizational feat, since it involved special manufacture and distribution (including during holidays) of over 100 food products. Daily consumption of xylitol was about 50 g per person. When pre-cavitation carious lesions were included in the caries score, the caries increment was zero in the xylitol group.

Since then a number of clinical trials have been conducted of daily use of xylitol products in addition to a usual sugar-containing diet—either partial substitution or supplementation. Evidence is sufficiently strong to conclude that xylitol is non-cariogenic. A more interesting discussion concerns the anti-cariogenic role of xylitol and this has been investigated by many people. There is good evidence that the ability of plaque to produce acids by metabolism of sugars is reduced by xylitol. This seems to be explained adequately by the differential decrease in *Streptococcus mutans* in plaque exposed to xylitol and, possibly, in a decrease in plaque quantity. Although xylitol is toxic to some strains of oral streptococci, the practical effect of this toxicity has yet to be demonstrated. Several long-term studies have indicated that adaptation by plaque organisms to metabolize xylitol is very unlikely.

## Hydrogenated glucose syrup (Lycasin)

Lycasin is the registered trade name for hydrogenated glucose syrup, which is obtained by enzymatic hydrolysis of starch. Lycasin syrup is an aqueous solution of sorbitol (about 7 per cent), hydrogenated oligosaccharides, and polysaccharides. It is important to differentiate between hydrogenated glucose syrup, which is sugar-free, and glucose syrup, which is basically a solution of glucose.

## Isomalt (Palatinit)

Palatinit is the registered trade name of isomalt which is an equimolar mixture of two disaccharide alcohols; this is sometimes shortened to 'GPS + GPM'. The first report of the potential use of isomalt as a non-cariogenic sweetener dates back to the 1970s.

# Intense sweeteners

Because of their composition, intense sweeteners are very unlikely to promote dental caries and research has been directed at investigating the caries-inhibitory properties of these substances. Each will be discussed briefly.

**Saccharin** was first discovered in 1879 and has been used widely as a food additive for more than 80 years. Saccharin is 300 times sweeter than sucrose. It has a bitter taste in concentrations over 0.1 per cent although the degree of appreciation of bitterness varies considerably between people. It is used as a table-top sweetener and extensively in soft drinks. Saccharin is absorbed and excreted (almost wholly in the urine) without being metabolized. For an equivalent amount of sweetness, it is much cheaper than sugar.

**Acesulfame K** was discovered in 1967 by Hoechst AG, Germany. It is known by the trade name Sunett and is approximately 130 times sweeter than sucrose. It has a clean sweet taste and is stable in aqueous solutions over a wide pH range and can withstand moderately severe heat treatment. It is thought to have a good potential as a sweetener in most classes of foods and drinks. It is not metabolized and is excreted unchanged (mainly via the urine).

**Aspartame** is a dipeptide consisting of aspartic acid and phenylalanine. It is approximately 200 times sweeter than sucrose with a similar taste to sucrose. It is manufactured by G D Searle under the trade names Canderel and NutraSweet. It is moderately stable in solution although prolonged heat treatment and storage hastens its breakdown with subsequent loss of sweetness. It is now used extensively in soft drinks. It is digested as a protein and its metabolism is similar to that of dietary phenylalanine and aspartic acid. Ingestion of aspartame should be avoided by individuals with phenylketonuria (PKU) (approximately 1 in 10 000 live births) who have a genetic defect of phenylalanine metabolism.

There is some evidence that saccharin inhibits bacterial growth and metabolism, and one study has shown that the addition of saccharin to the diet of rats resulted in less caries development. However, this was not duplicated in another study and the practical significance of these results is unclear. The other intense sweeteners appear to have no direct effect on caries development.

# Sugarless chewing gums

The growth in the use of sugarless chewing gums has been a great success story. There is now considerable evidence that their use positively benefits dental health. In 1987, sugarless gums had only about 17 per cent of the UK chewing gum market; this rose to 60 per cent by 1995.

There are perhaps four scientific aspects to consider:

(1) the effects of sugared gum;

## Box 3.10 Relative costs of non-sugar sweeteners

| Sucrose | 1 |
|---------|---|
| Sorbitol | 2 |
| Maltitol | 4 |
| Xylitol | 6 |

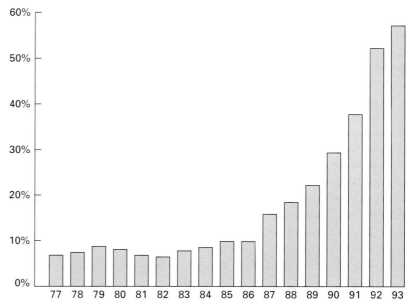

**Figure 3.17** The percentage share of the UK chewing gum market held by sugar-free gums, between 1977 and 1993. Data from The Wrigley Company with permission.

(2) the benefits of sugarless gum;

(3) whether xylitol gums are better than sorbitol gums; and

(4) whether polyols can be combined with other preventive agents to provide extra benefit.

## Effect of sugared gum and dental caries

There have been at least seven trials comparing the effect on dental caries development of sugared gum versus no gum. In five of these trials, the subjects using sugared gum developed more caries than those not using any gum, while in another two trials, caries development in the subjects in the sugared gum and no gum groups was similar. Thus, there is no evidence that chewing sugared gum benefits dental health; on the contrary, it appears to increase caries development.

## Dental benefits of sugarless gum

There have been at least ten clinical trials of the dental benefits of chewing sugarless gum. In some of these trials, sugarless gum has been tested against sugared gum. The results of these trials showed that substitution of non-sugar sweeteners for sugar in chewing gums resulted in substantial caries reductions. In the other trials, the test group chewed sugarless gum but the control group did not chew any gum at all. Caries development was less in the test group compared with the control group. These results were important as they showed that chewing sugarless gum actually helped prevent caries—probably by encouraging healing of very early carious lesions through increased salivary flow.

## Superiority of xylitol

The third question—is xylitol better than other polyols in chewing gum—was answered in what is called the Belize study—a 40 month double-blind longitudinal study which was carried out between 1989 and 1993 in Belize, central America, involving nine groups of children. It was concluded that

- xylitol gums were more effective than sorbitol gums in caries prevention;
- chewing five times rather than three times per day was more effective;
- mixtures of xylitol and sorbitol were less effective in preventing caries than xylitol alone, but more effective than sorbitol alone;
- sorbitol gum provided some caries-preventive effect, while sugared gum increased caries development;
- caries reductions were observed in primary and permanent teeth, and hardening of carious lesions was recorded in groups using the polyol gums.

## Benefits of combination with polyols

The fourth question concerns the possible additive effects of polyols and other preventive agents. Chewing gums have been used as vehicles for many anti-caries agents, such as fluoride, phosphate salts, and carbamide, and other therapeutic agents, such as antibiotics, chlorhexidine, and antiseptics. As yet, data are insufficient to conclude that any of these additives have any extra caries-preventive effect, although trends in that direction have been observed.

It is not surprising that in the light of the very favourable results of clinical trials of sugarless chewing gums, and xylitol gums in particular, public health authorities have encouraged their use. An example of such a campaign in Finland is described in Chapter 9.

# Toothfriendly sweets and product accreditation

Over 20 years ago, the dental benefits of non-sugar sweeteners was apparent. In Switzerland, this led to a partnership between the dental profession and industry to launch the 'toothfriendly' idea. This has been a great success in Switzerland and there are now similar organizations in seven other countries, including the UK. In addition to the toothfriendly idea, the British Dental Association has recently introduced accreditation for foods and drinks. Both of these aspects are considered further in Chapter 9.

# Medicines

The volume of liquid oral medicines consumed, often by children, is considerable. For example, ten million litres of liquid oral medicines were dispensed in the UK in 1987, the majority sugar-based. A number of studies have related the

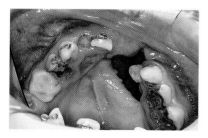

**Figure 3.18** Extensive caries in the primary dentition of a child with a cleft of the primary and secondary palate with a history of frequent use of sweetened liquid oral medicines.

**Summary of investigations for anti-caries properties**

| | |
|---|---|
| 1920s | Vitamin D investigated for its anti-caries properties |
| Early 1930s | Fluorides |
| Late 1930s | Substances in unrefined cereals |
| 1950s | Phosphates |
| 1970s | Cheese and components of milk Salivary stimulants |

frequent use of sugar-containing liquid oral medicines to caries development: this is particularly depressing as it is most often chronically ill children who have to take these medicines, for whom dental disease and dental care could be an additional burden (Fig. 3.18). A number of UK health education campaigns have urged prescribers and purchasers to switch from sugar-containing to sugar-free medicines. These have been moderately successful, but still only between 30 and 40 per cent of liquid oral medicines dispensed are presently sugar-free in the UK.

# Protective factors in foods

For nearly 100 years, dental research workers have been searching for components in foods which protect teeth against caries development—could it be that the rise in caries prevalence over the past 100 years has not been due solely to the increased consumption of sugars, but because food refinement has removed caries protective factors from the diet? This is difficult to answer with any certainty, as we shall see. Moving on from this argument, if any protective factors were isolated, could these be added to our cariogenic diet to reduce the risk of caries? Taken to its limit this might involve, for example, adding fluoride to sugar in order to reduce the cariogenicity of sugar. This particular example is unlikely to be accepted because of the uncontrolled use of this fortified sugar would risk excessive fluoride ingestion.

# Protective factors in plants

The observations of Osborn and colleagues that South African Bantu had a very low prevalence of dental caries despite a high carbohydrate diet began the search for components of the human diet which may protect teeth against dental caries. Since then, many possible protective factors in plant foods, not necessarily normal constituents, have been studied. One of the groups studied by Osborn were workers in sugar plantations who, in Osborn's survey, had lower dental caries experience than would be expected from the large quantities of sugars consumed. The results of other surveys of dental health of sugar cane chewers in Africa and the Caribbean have, though, been equivocal.

The early work in South Africa led others to try to identify protective factors in plant foods. This was the birth of extensive research into **organic phosphates**. Separate from this line, but progressing in parallel with it, have been the many investigations into the caries-preventive potential of **inorganic phosphates**—the origins of this line of research go back to the days of Mellanby and her 'calcifying factors', as discussed in Chapter 2. While inorganic calcium and phosphates are considered to act through a common ion effect, organic phosphates act in an entirely different way, by being adsorbed on to the surface of enamel. The evidence concerning the effectiveness of protective factors comes from three main sources—animal experiments, laboratory experiments, and human clinical trials.

The very great research activity in this field is illustrated by the observation that by the mid-1960s, results of over 100 rat experiments on this topic had been published. There was no doubt that adding inorganic phosphates to the cariogenic diet of rats decreased caries development. Sodium salts were more effective than calcium salts, probably because calcium salts are less soluble. A number of human clinical trials were conducted, adding inorganic phosphates to chewing gum, cereals, and the general diet, but the results were disappointing. The reasons why inorganic phosphates were effective in rats, but not in man, is not entirely clear, but it has been suggested that saliva is more highly saturated in phosphate in humans than in rats, allowing more scope for additional phosphate to act in rats. However, it is difficult to reconcile this viewpoint entirely since it is accepted that part of the explanation for the non-cariogenicity of cow's milk is its high calcium and phosphate content.

The story with organic phosphate compounds is rather similar. Calcium sucrose phosphate was marketed for many years in Australia as a caries-preventive additive, but clinical trial evidence did not support its continued use. The most promising of the organic phosphates was phytate, identified as the most active substance in unrefined cereals. The effectiveness of phytate appears to be due to its ability to adsorb readily and firmly to enamel surfaces and so prevent the dissolution of enamel by acid. It was certainly effective at preventing caries when added powdered to the diets of rats. However, the problem was that it was present naturally inside the bran particles and so was not readily available in its natural form, in unrefined foods, in the mouth. This line of research declined when it was realized that phytate reduced the absorption of dietary calcium, magnesium, iron, and zinc from the gut and, although humans can adapt to increased levels of phytate and restore their level of absorption of calcium at least, it is probable that this side-effect will make it unwise to recommend the use of phytate as a food additive.

**Honey** is unlikely to be less cariogenic than refined sugars (Fig. 3.19). Theoretically black treacle could be less cariogenic because of its high calcium content (0.5 per cent), but this has not been established.

The results of the clinical trial carried out at the Vipeholm Hospital in Sweden in the 1940s and 50s suggested that chocolate may be less cariogenic than sugar confectionery. This led to speculation that **chocolate** might contain a protective factor. The active ingredient (known as 'cocoa-factor') was isolated, but the extraction was expensive and it was considered that using this cocoa factor as a method of dental caries prevention would be less efficient than the use of fluoride.

Likewise, the major constituent of **liquorice**—glycyrrhizinic acid—has a potential caries-preventive property. However, it does have undesirable properties of strong taste, dark staining, and, more importantly, it disturbs the electrolyte balance in the body, so its usefulness as a dietary additive is, therefore, very limited.

There has been remarkably little research into the effect of fibre (now known by nutritionists as non-starch polysaccharide, NSP) and dental caries. For years, people have assumed that fibrous foods clean the teeth by physical action, stimulate helpful salivary flow, and improve gingival health by stimulating the gingivae. There has been more research on this latter aspect in relation to gingival health than dental caries, and the conclusions are that fibrous foods probably

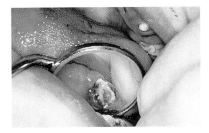

**Figure 3.19** Gross caries of a mandibular second primary molar tooth in a 16 month old Siamese twin whose mother was advised by staff on the hospital ward to dip the baby's dummy in honey to pacify her.

have little influence on gingival health in humans. Chewing affects salivary flow in two ways: first, there is an immediate response of increased salivary flow and, second, there is a long-term increase in resting and stimulated flow rates. Both are important. The lower dental caries experience observed by some epidemiologists in sugar cane chewers, described above, has been considered to be due to possible protective factors and/or increased salivary flow. The latter explanation seems the more likely.

## Milk and dairy products

The non-cariogenicity of cow's milk has been discussed already. The high calcium and phosphate content and the low cariogenicity of lactose are accepted as likely explanations. Fats, proteins, and the phosphoprotein casein, present in milk, have been considered as caries preventive but they are probably less important than the minerals.

Fats aid oral clearance of foods—which may be another reason for the suggested lower cariogenicity of chocolate compared with sugar confectionery. Proteins adsorb onto tooth surfaces and could, in theory, decrease caries risk—but precise evidence is lacking. The anti-caries role of casein has been investigated fairly extensively, principally in Australia. It is certainly effective when added to cariogenic diets of rats. Casein has a number of advantages as an additive, being commercially available, nutritive, and relatively inexpensive, but the palatability of casein-enhanced chocolate was unacceptable in clinical trials. Further work has investigated certain phosphopeptides, which are components of casein, for their anti-caries action: these have an acceptable taste but, as yet, there is a lack of data to support their use.

The possible anti-caries role of vitamin D was discussed in Chapter 2. Originally, it was assumed that any role would be pre-eruptive. However, some of the observed effects must have been post-eruptive, but data are very limited and vitamin D's role in caries prevention remains an enigma.

## Fluoride

Fluoride is the most important caries-protective agent. Its wide and effective use is one of the great success stories in preventive medicine. Water is the most important dietary vehicle for fluorides but fluoride is also effective when added to salt, milk, or given as drops and tablets (so-called fluoride dietary supplements).

On a worldwide public health basis, the addition of fluoride to toothpastes is the single most effective method of topical caries prevention. Other ways of applying fluoride therapeutically include mouth rinses, gels, and varnishes, but consideration of these is outside the scope of this book.

The use of fluoride is equated so strongly with the prevention of dental caries that it is sometimes difficult to appreciate that the early history (the first 30 years of this century) of fluorides and teeth concerned mottling of dental enamel. It was not until the publication of the extensive epidemiological surveys by H. Trendley Dean in 1942 of the dental health of 12–14 year old children in 21 cities in the USA that the strength of the relationship between the concentration of fluoride in drinking water and experience of dental caries was clearly established. The optimum level of fluoride in drinking water was set at 1 part per million or 1 mg F/l water as the best balance between dental caries and dental fluorosis, based on the considerable amount of epidemiological data and, on 25 January 1945, sodium fluoride was added to the water supply of the city of Grand Rapids, Michigan. So began an era of **water fluoridation**, a vitally important public health measure, which now reaches at least 210 million people worldwide. The effectiveness of fluoridation has been monitored in many communities and, in 24 studies of primary teeth, the modal percentage caries reduction has been between 40 and 50 per cent; for permanent teeth, the modal percentage caries reduction has been 50–60 per cent in 33 studies (Fig. 3.20). These results are in line with the oft-quoted statement that fluoridation cuts caries by half.

**Salt** is the second most important dietary vehicle for ensuring adequate ingestion of fluoride. Fluoridated salt has been on sale in Switzerland since 1955. Even by 1983 it was available in 23 Swiss cantons and used by 73 per cent of the population. The fluoride concentration is 250 mg F/kg salt. Its use has spread to central and south America and it is especially useful in areas which lack public water supplies.

**Milk** has been considered as a possible vehicle for fluoride for at least 30 years. All the results of the trials of fluoridated milk have shown substantial caries preventive effects, especially when milk consumption begins before the eruption of permanent teeth.

During the early years of water fluoridation, it was recognized that fluoride in the form of **tablets** might be a sensible alternative when fluoridation of water was not feasible. Since the result of the first trial of fluoride tablets was published in the USA, over 50 trials have been reported: caries reductions have been substantial.

The appropriate use of fluorides has brought great benefits to very large numbers of people throughout the world. Too little fluoride increases the risk of caries development, but too much fluoride can be detrimental. In Chapter 2, the ability of excessive ingestion of fluoride to cause dental enamel opacities was emphasized. The appropriate use of fluoride is vital, and readers are referred to more comprehensive texts such as Murray (1996) or Rugg-Gunn (1993) given in the list of further reading.

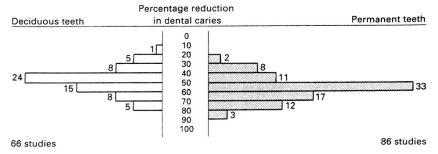

**Figure 3.20** Percentage reductions in dental caries observed in 113 studies into the effectiveness of artificial water fluoridation in 23 countries. Sixty-six studies gave results for the deciduous dentition and 86 studies gave results for the permanent dentition. Source: Murray *et al.* (1991).

# Salivary stimulants

The pH of unstimulated (resting) saliva is around 7.0 but rises rapidly to pH 8.0 or higher when flow rate increases (Fig. 3.21).

This fast flow of saliva will help to remove food and degradation products such as acid; the high pH will help to neutralize acids in plaque; and the high levels of calcium and phosphate will aid remineralization of any demineralized enamel (Fig. 3.22). Although the physiology has been known for many years, the realization of the potential importance of this method of caries control is fairly recent. Its greatest success has been the now well established caries-preventive effect of sugarless chewing gum. There is a dose–response relationship, since the caries-preventive effect increases as the frequency of chewing gum per day increases.

Other components of our diet are also powerful salivary stimulants. Part of the favourable action of cheese is likely to be due to the fast flow of saliva induced by chewing sharp-tasting cheese. It would seem logical that chewing fibrous sugar-free foods will help to control dental caries. This has already been considered in relation to sugar cane, but this subject has been under-researched.

# Summary

- The way dental caries occurs is now well known. In simple terms, sugars in the mouth are converted by bacteria in dental plaque to acids which dissolve the mineral of enamel beneath the plaque. The carious lesion is initially sub-surface. The surface, although with slightly reduced mineral content, is intact and the lesion looks like a white spot (Fig. 3.22). It is vitally important to recognize this pre-cavitation stage—it is a danger sign—as it can remineralize if given a chance. A change in diet, fluoride therapy, and plaque removal are all important.

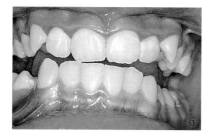

**Figure 3.22** Precavitation carious lesions which will remineralize, if conditions are favourable.

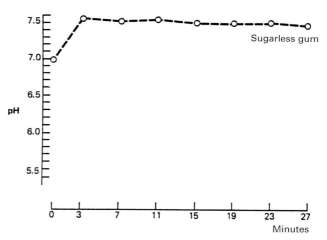

**Figure 3.21** Stephan curve produced by sugarless chewing gum. The rise in plaque pH can be seen clearly.

- Dietary carbohydrates consist basically of sugars and starch. There is no doubt that sugars cause caries; starch can cause caries but much less so than sugars. Of the common dietary sugars, lactose is the least cariogenic. No sugar has been shown to be more cariogenic than sucrose.

- There is little evidence that fresh fruit and vegetables cause dental caries, although sugar-containing fruit-flavoured drinks, when fed frequently in bottles or reservoir feeders and especially when given as comforters, are a major cause of caries in infants and young children.

- Milk is not cariogenic, although rarely caries occurs in children breastfed on demand for many years.

- Staple starchy foods such as potatoes, rice, pasta, and bread are not seen as significant causes of caries. When starchy foods are heat-treated and finely ground, as happens in many snack foods, shorter chain saccharides are formed which are more available to salivary amylase and plaque bacteria and thus have potential for caries development. Advances in food technology have led to an increase in the number of short-chain saccharides in processed foods made from staple starchy foods. The cariogenicity of these foods is likely to be between the cariogenicities of sugars and starch.

- Advances in food technology and the appreciation that sugars cause caries have also led to an expansion in the availability and use of non-sugar sweeteners. Bulk sweeteners are used mainly in confectionery, chewing gums, and liquid oral medicines, while intense sweeteners are used mainly in drinks and for enhancing the flavour of chewing gums and other foods and medicines. Substitution of these sweeteners for sugars will benefit dental health. The greatest success so far has been in the sugar-free chewing gum market; there is no doubt that chewing sugar-free gum benefits dental health.

- Some components of our diet can protect against dental caries. The most important of these are fluoride and sugar-free salivary stimulants. Phosphates, both inorganic and organic, have been investigated very extensively but are unlikely to become caries-preventive food additives.

- How and when foods are eaten has an important influence on caries development. There is much evidence that frequent eating of sugary foods is particularly dangerous. Frequent eating prolongs the time plaque pH is low, encouraging demineralization, and decreases the time that plaque pH is high, when remineralization can occur. Although frequency of intake is very important, the amount of sugar consumed is also independently a relevant factor. How these conclusions can be brought together in effective practical advice will be considered in Chapters 7 to 10.

# Further reading

Downer, M. C. (1998). The changing pattern of dental disease over 50 years. *Br. Dent. J.* 185, 36–41.

Edgar, W. M. (1998). Sugar substitutes, chewing gum and dental caries—a review. *Br. Dent. J.* 184, 29–32.

Lennon, M. A. and Beal, J. F. (eds) (1996). Proceedings of the international symposium on water fluoridation. *Community Dental Health* **13** (Suppl. 2), 1–71.

Moynihan, P. J. (1995). The relationship between diet, nutrition and dental health: an overview and update for the 1990s. *Nutr. Res. Rev.* **8**, 193–224.

Moynihan, P. J. (1998). Update on the nomenclature of carbohydrates and their dental effects. *J. Dent.* **26**, 209–18.

Murray, J. J. (ed) (1996) *The prevention of oral disease*, Oxford University Press, Oxford.

Rugg-Gunn, A. J. (1993). *Nutrition and dental health*, Chapters 5–10. Oxford University Press, Oxford.

# 4

# Diet and dental erosion

# Diet and dental erosion

Journal of Dentistry, 2, 85–88

## Fruit juice erosion—an increasing danger?

R. S. Levine, B.Ch.D., Ph.D., L.D.S.R.C.S.(Eng.)
*Department of Oral Medicine, Turner Dental School, Manchester*

**ABSTRACT**

Two cases of fruit juice erosion of teeth are described and the differential diagnosis of erosion, abrasion, attrition, and arrested caries is discussed. Individuals susceptible to erosion are defined on the basis of fluid intake and salivary gland function. Attention is drawn to evidence of a fourfold increase in fruit juice consumption since 1956 and the possibility is raised that this may result in an

This form of erosion has been reported by Darby (1892), and Miller (1907) and in Sicilian lemon suckers by Pickerill (1912). More recently cases have been reported by Lovestedt (1944), Stafne and Lovestedt (1947), Hicks (1950), James and Parfitt (1953), Finch, (1957), and Allen (1967). The erosive property of acid beverages has been confirmed using laboratory

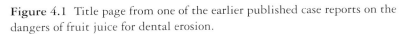

**Figure 4.1** Title page from one of the earlier published case reports on the dangers of fruit juice for dental erosion.

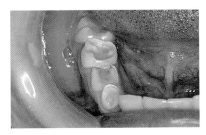

**Figure 4.2** Extensive loss of tooth tissue in the lower right primary canine and molar teeth as a consequence of food-acid-associated erosion.

This prophetic article appeared in the *Journal of Dentistry* in 1973, describing erosion of dental enamel in two young female patients, the first of whom drank the juice of six oranges each day, while the second consumed the juice of ten oranges as well as eating two whole oranges or apples and stewed rhubarb each day. It seems that Dr Levine was right: fresh fruit and fruit juices were becoming more available. In addition, the media was making a thin figure desirable (Fig. 4.3). By the end of that decade, caries prevalence and severity were declining in the UK and many other developed countries, and there was more chance that a dentist and patient would notice loss of dental enamel from other causes—one of which was erosion. Thirty years ago, dental epidemiological surveys were largely interested in recording dental caries, as this disease dominated dentistry; now, developmental defects of enamel and dental erosion have become important. Erosion can be difficult and expensive to treat—early recognition and prevention is the goal.

## Are the prevalence and severity of erosion really increasing?

There is a perception that they are. People point to the great rise in soft drink consumption (an 800 per cent increase since the 1950s; Fig. 4.4) which is strongly suspected of being a prime cause of erosion.

Other people point to the increased prevalence of anorexia nervosa and bulimia, which now affect about 5 per cent of young women aged 20–30 years in western industrialized countries.

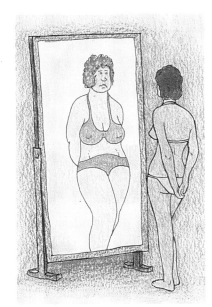

**Figure 4.3** A disordered body image is a feature of eating disorders.

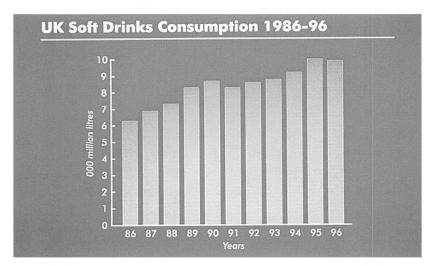

Figure 4.4  The change in soft drinks consumption in the UK 1986–96.
Source: British Soft Drinks Association/Zenith International.

The truth is, we do not know for certain that the prevalence of erosion is increasing as there have not yet been any repeated epidemiological surveys. In fact, the first epidemiological survey was published in 1991: this took place in Switzerland where 391 adults aged between 26 and 50 years were examined in their homes. Twelve per cent of the younger age group (26–30 years) and 10 per cent of the older age group (31–50 years) had some erosion on buccal and lingual surfaces of teeth. Eight per cent of the younger age group and 13 per cent of the older age group had severe erosion on these tooth surfaces. Thirty per cent and 43 per cent in the two age groups, respectively, had severe erosion of occlusal surfaces.

This was followed by a survey of over a thousand 14 year old children in north-west England published in 1993. Thirty-one per cent of the children had exposed dentine but this was mainly on the incisal edge; 8 per cent of children had exposed dentine on occlusal and or lingual surfaces. One year later, a survey of erosion in 4–5 year old children living in the West Midlands, England, showed that nearly half the children were affected.

In 1992/3, the first of the National Diet and Nutrition Surveys in mainland UK was carried out. This survey was undertaken on children aged 1.5–4.5 years. This included a survey of oral health which was the first to assess the prevalence of dental erosion nationally. For all ages combined, nearly 10 per cent had erosion involving the dentine on the palatal surfaces of upper primary incisors. National surveys of child dental health in the UK have taken place every 10 years since 1973. The 1993 survey was the first of these to record dental erosion: the buccal and lingual surfaces of maxillary incisors were examined. Half of the children aged 5 years had eroded primary teeth and, in a quarter of children, erosion had reached the dentine and, in some cases, involved the pulp. By the age of 14 years, nearly 30 per cent had some erosion into dentine.

We have to wait for such surveys to be repeated to have a clear idea of whether the prevalence of erosion is changing in the UK.

## Case report

Rosy, an anorexic patient in her late 30s, consumed a bizarre diet, a page of which is reproduced in Fig 4.5. Analysis of her diet revealed that consumption of vitamin A was seven times, calcium five times, and oxalate eight times the recommended daily intake. The combination of the latter two is likely to lead to formation of calcium oxalate and the deposition of stones in body organs. The effects on her dentition can be seen in Figs 4.6 and 4.7. The slow nature of the process has not led to any symptoms although the buccal erosion cavities have been restored previously with glass–ionomer cements.

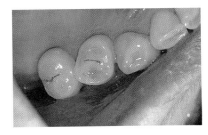

**Figure** 4.6 Wear into dentine involving the incisal and occlusal surfaces of the remaining permanent teeth of the patient whose diet is given in Fig. 4.5.

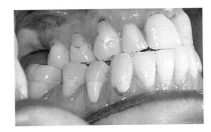

**Figure** 4.7 Wear of the buccal coronal and root surfaces in the same patient as Fig. 4.6, much of which has been restored.

DAY: ...Monday...................

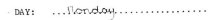

| TIME | FOOD | QUANTITY |
|------|------|----------|
| | Ginseng | 500 mg |
| 6 am | 6 fluid oz of fresh orange juice | 6 fluid oz |
| | Apples | 3/4 lb |
| | Cheese | 3 oz |
| | 6 cups of coffee with 5 oz milk | |
| 12 – 1 pm | Corned beef | 3½ oz |
| | Cabbage | 2 oz |
| | Parsnip | 6 oz |
| | Carrots | 6 oz |
| | Onion | 2 oz |
| | Rhubarb | 3/4 lb |
| | 4 cups of coffee with 3½ oz milk | |
| 4 pm | Cheese | 3 oz |
| | Apples | 3/4 lb |
| | 4 cups of coffee + milk | |
| | Ginseng | 500 mg |
| 10 30pm | 4 cups of coffee + milk | |
| | Total fruit | |
| | 2¼ lbs + 6 fluid oz orange juice | |

**Figure** 4.5  A typical day in the diet of this anorexic patient.

## What is erosion?

Erosion is defined as the 'physical result of a pathological, chronic, localised, painless (initially) loss of dental hard tissue which is chemically etched away from the tooth surface by acid and/or chelation without bacterial involvement'.

This definition emphasizes the slow insidious nature of erosion which rarely causes discomfort until advanced, when the person affected becomes conscious of sensitivity to temperature and/or sweetness. It emphasizes that the acids responsible for erosion do not come from bacterial fermentation of dietary sugars—which is the principal factor in dental caries aetiology. The tooth surfaces affected by erosion and dental caries are very different. Caries occurs beneath plaque, and plaque can be found in areas that are difficult to clean well, namely in the pits and fissures, on approximal surfaces between teeth, and more rarely, around the gingival margin of the teeth. Erosion occurs in areas free from plaque but exposed to acids—the palatal and buccal surfaces of incisors, the occlusal cusps, and the palatal and buccal surfaces of posterior teeth.

Erosion can be confused with two other causes of tooth wear—abrasion and attrition. In Fig. 4.8 toothbrush abrasion has resulted in loss of enamel, exposing dentine on the buccal surfaces of teeth 43, 44. In Figs 4.9 and 4.10, tooth wear has affected the incisal edges of teeth 11, 21 as a consequence, primarily of the way the teeth occlude. In addition, erosion has produced some cupping of the incisal edges but also loss of enamel on the cuspal tips of the first premolars and palatal surfaces of the second premolar teeth. There is no doubt that much of tooth wear is combinations of erosion and abrasion or erosion and attrition. Enamel softened by acids may be brushed away with a toothbrush (this has been called abrasion) or worn away by mastication (which is called demastication). Although these three causes of tooth wear often occur in combination, in general, erosion is often seen in young people, while attrition is more common in older people.

## What causes erosion?

In broad terms, acids which cause erosion come from three sources—diet, the stomach, and the environment.

Dietary causes are listed in Table 4.1; this list includes medicaments. Not all of these are equally important, as will be discussed below.

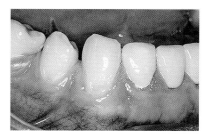

**Figure 4.8** Loss of buccal enamel as a consequence of toothbrush abrasion.

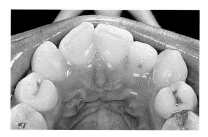

**Figure 4.9** Attrition of the incisal edges of the upper central incisors (teeth 11, 21).

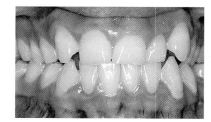

**Figure 4.10** The anterior occlusion of the patient in Fig. 4.9 showing the tooth-to-tooth contact of the upper and lower incisor teeth.

Box 4.1  Non-carious forms of tooth wear

| Erosion | Chemical etching and dissolution |
|---|---|
| Abrasion | Mechanical wear by means of other objects (e.g. toothbrush, hairpins, etc.) |
| Attrition | Mechanical wear involving tooth-to-tooth contact |
| Demastication | Mechanical interaction between food and teeth |
| Abfraction | Wear as a consequence of tooth flexion from eccentric occlusal forces |
| Resorption | Wear of tooth tissue as a result of biological degradation |

Table 4.1.
Causes of erosion

| Diet | Medicaments |
|---|---|
| Acid carbonated beverages | Iron tonics |
| Citrus fruit juices and other acidic fruit juices | Liquid hydrochloric acid |
| Acidic un-carbonated beverages | Vitamin C |
| Acidic sport drinks | Aspirin |
| Wines | Acidic mouth-rinses |
| Cider | |
| Acidic herbal teas | |
| Citrus fruits | |
| Other acidic fruits and berries | |
| Salad dressing | |
| Vinegar conserves | |
| Acidic fruit-flavoured candies | |

## Case report

Margaret presented for an orthodontic assessment. It was noticed that she had severe wear involving her remaining primary teeth but without any symptoms (Fig. 4.11). Investigation of her diet revealed a frequent intake of fizzy drinks and fruit juice. Fortunately, the extensive wear of her primary teeth indicated the need to monitor this condition in the permanent teeth which, at the moment, show only minimal loss of enamel on the palatal surfaces of the upper incisors and occlusal surfaces of the first permanent molar teeth. Dietary advice was directed at confining fruit juice intake to a mealtime and limiting the use of fizzy drinks, even diet versions, to once or twice a week.

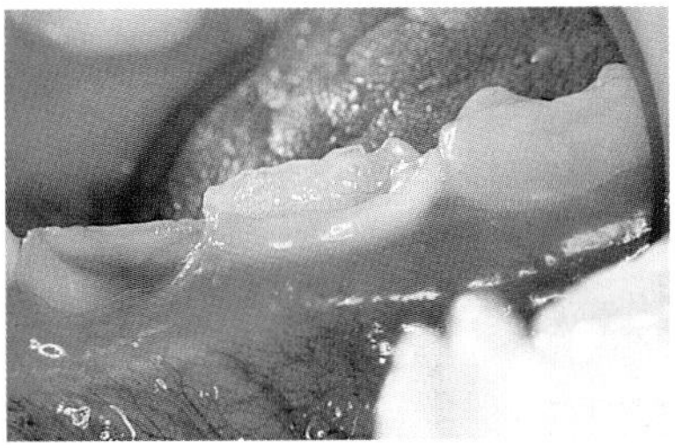

**Figure** 4.11 Severe wear of the lower primary first and second molar teeth.

Acids from the stomach are sometimes referred to as intrinsic acids. In broad terms, gastric acids may come to be in the mouth through vomiting or through

Table 4.2.
## Some causes of vomiting

Chronic gastritis
Intestinal obstruction
Migraine
Disturbances of labyrinthine
  apparatus
Pregnancy
Chemotherapeutic drugs
Alcoholism
Eating disorders

Table 4.3.
## Some causes of regurgitation or gastro-oesophageal reflex

Idiopathic
Impairment of gastro-oesophageal
  sphincter
Obesity
Pregnancy
After big meals

gastro-oesophageal reflux and regurgitation. Vomiting is the forceful expulsion of gastric contents through the mouth and is a common manifestation of many chronic and psychosomatic disorders (Table 4.2). Regurgitation and reflux of gastric contents into the mouth are generally seen with gastro-oesophageal incompetence, with increased gastric pressures, or with increased gastric volume (Table 4.3). Rumination, where the gastric contents are regurgitated, re-chewed and re-swallowed, is rare in humans. The severity of erosion will depend very much on the frequency of vomiting or regurgitation and the length of time that it continues. For example, vomiting during pregnancy is unlikely to lead to severe erosion, while frequent and continued vomiting in anorexia nervosa, bulimia nervosa, or alcoholism often leads to severe erosion. Gastro-oesophageal reflux disease (GORD) is often 'silent', in that the person affected is unaware that it occurs. In one survey, 2 per cent of normal individuals refluxed at least once per month. Upon questioning, they may be aware of occasionally having a bad taste in their mouth, for example, upon waking.

## Case report

Stuart had cancer as a small child and one of the consequences of his chemotherapy and radiotherapy was to reduce salivary gland function. In addition, the disease, and perhaps its treatment, has resulted in swallowing difficulties. His mother operates an ice-cream van which Stuart has easy access to! Caries of first permanent molars was a consequence which resulted in early loss of these teeth. Now he has a problem with wear (Fig. 4.12). Salivary flow appeared to be a little diminished and there were no dietary causal factors identified in a 3 day dietary record. Subsequent monitoring of the reflux of gastric contents with a pH probe passed down the oesophagus (Fig. 4.13) for 18 h showed there to be significant reflux (Fig. 4.14) which resolved with appropriate drug therapy (Fig. 4.15). In Stuart's case, as with many people, there was a variety of factors operating: diminished buffering by saliva, gastro-oesophageal reflux, and perhaps more to his diet than he was prepared to admit. These together caused a significant amount of tooth tissue loss, making repair of the sensitive teeth difficult, particularly until these factors had been isolated and modified.

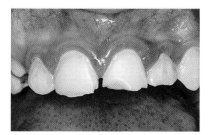

**Figure** 4.12 Extensive wear of the erupted permanent teeth, especially the upper incisors, in a 12 year old boy.

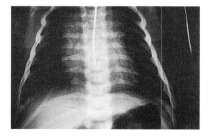

**Figure** 4.13 pH monitoring within the oesophagus in order to diagnose gastro-oesophageal reflux.

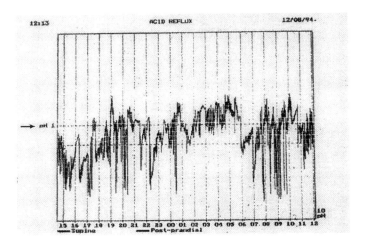

**Figure** 4.14  A trace from the pH monitoring indicating frequent periods when the pH in the oesophagus dropped below a critical level (indicated by the arrow) indicative of reflux of gastric acid.

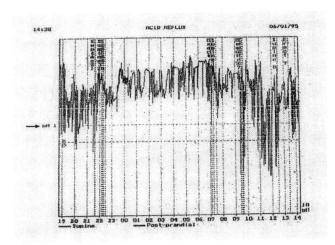

**Figure** 4.15  A similar trace recorded after the patient had received appropriate drug therapy for his reflux showing the pH in the oesophagus maintained well above the critical level (indicated by the arrow), apart from periods when the patient was supine.

The third source of acids which causes dental erosion is the environment (Table 4.4). Improvements in industrial hygiene have meant that these causes are now rare in industrial countries. The addition of chlorine gas to swimming pools makes the water acid: this is usually neutralized satisfactorily but occasionally errors occur and the acidic water causes erosion to the teeth of competitive swimmers.

Table 4.4.
Environmental
(occupational) causes of
erosion

| |
| --- |
| Battery factory workers |
| Workers in zinc galvanising factories |
| Workers exposed to etching and cleaning processes involving acids |
| Professional wine tasters |
| Competitive swimmers |

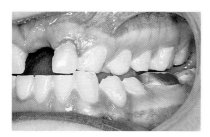

**Figure** 4.16 A combination of factors have led to substantial tooth tissue loss in this patient who is a trainee welder. This includes the loss of a central incisor tooth, replaced now by a resin-retained bridge.

## Case report

Karl took up an apprenticeship as a trainee welder. The work was hot and claustrophobic—working behind a mask with protective workwear left him thirsty, and the temptation to leave off the mask on occasions was strong. The environment in a welding shed can produce erosive gases. In Karl's case, he drank large quantities of fizzy drinks to slake his thirst. The combined effects of frequent, low pH drinks and an acidic working environment resulted in considerable tooth wear (Fig. 4.16). Once these factors had been identified, the affected surfaces could be covered and protected without the likelihood of further tooth destruction around the restorations.

Although intrinsic and environmental causes are clinically important, this book is mostly concerned with dietary causes. The evidence relating dietary acids and eating habits to dental erosion comes from several types of study: case reports, epidemiological studies, experimental clinical studies, animal experiments, and *in vitro* investigations. These will now be reviewed to see what lessons can be learnt.

### Case reports

Most of the clinical evidence linking specific dietary factors to dental erosion comes from anecdotal case reports. These include

- marked erosion within 3 months of drinking lemon juice daily 'for therapeutic reasons';
- marked erosion of the labial surfaces of upper front teeth from daily sucking of segments of lemon;
- erosion in a lady with diabetes insipidus who drank much fruit juices and fruit-flavoured cordials each day;
- severe erosion in a young man who had the habit of holding a cola drink in his mouth because he enjoyed the feeling of bubbles in his mouth;
- severe erosion in a youth who consumed nearly 2 litres of a diet cola drink per day for 2 years;
- severe erosion was seen on the occlusal surfaces of maxillary and mandibular teeth of a middle-aged lady who chewed vitamin C tablets (ascorbic acid) three times a day for 3 years (the erosion was mainly on the side of her mouth used for chewing);
- similar erosion has been related to chewing of aspirin (acetylsalicylic acid) tablets.

Several authors have recommended that acid beverages should be drunk through a straw. However, there are case reports of severe erosion of maxillary incisor teeth where the child held the straw against the labial surfaces of these teeth (Fig. 4.17) . The same condition has been reported when the spout of drinking cups and the teat of infant comforters are placed between the lips but not between the teeth.

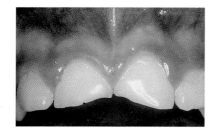

**Figure** 4.17 Loss of enamel from the labial surface of the maxillary central incisor teeth as a result of drinking fizzy drinks with a straw held against the labial surface of the incisors.

## Epidemiological studies

There have been a small number of epidemiological surveys which have not only recorded prevalence (see above) but also related prevalence to possible causative factors recorded by questionnaire or interview. The accuracy of some of the responses can be questioned and sometimes habits change, so that it is not surprising that often relationships between possible causative factors and erosion are weak. One of the most thoroughly analysed studies was a case–control study conducted in Finland (Table 4.5). One hundred and six patients with erosion were identified and paired with 100 controls who were randomly selected from the same population but who were free from erosion; the mean age of the groups was 33 and 36 years. Diet was the factor associated with erosion in 32 cases, gastric symptoms in another 27, and both of these factors in 46 cases. No risk factor could be identified in one case. Of the dietary risk factors, the following were ranked in order of occurrence in the case subjects (with the number of cases in brackets):

- citrus fruits (53)
- other fruits (42)
- soft drinks (32)
- sports drinks (8)
- pickles (4)
- apple vinegar (9).

  Similar information for gastric symptoms (at least once a week) was

- vomiting (12)
- sour taste (32)

Table 4.5.
Factors associated with dental erosion (106 cases and 100 controls: adult dental patients in Helsinki, Finland)

| | Adjusted odds ratio | Population attributable risk (%) |
|---|---|---|
| Citrus fruits (more than twice a day) | 37 | 26 |
| Vomiting (weekly or more often) | 31 | 23 |
| Other gastric symptoms (weekly or more often) | 10 | 67 |
| Apple vinegar (weekly or more often) | 10 | 15 |
| Soft drinks (4–6 or more per week) | 4 | 26 |
| Sport drinks (weekly or more often) | 4 | 15 |
| Saliva flow, unstimulated (< 0.1 ml/min) | 5 | 19 |

Jarvinen *et al.* (1991).

- belching (28)
- heartburn (30)
- stomach-ache (34)
- pain on awakening (8).

The relative importance of association between erosion and all the different risk factors was determined using multivariate analyses to compute adjusted odds ratios. These are given in Table 4.5 along with the population attributable risk, which is the percentage decrease in occurrence of dental erosion in the population which would occur if that causative factor was eliminated. For example, if sports drinks were not used and other risk factors were not increased, the prevalence of erosion would decline by 15 per cent. The odds ratio indicates that, for example, people having sports drinks weekly or more often are four times more likely to have some erosion than people not having sports drinks weekly or more often. This table clearly indicates the degree of risk for each factor and the benefits which could accrue to the population from its elimination.

In the UK 1992–3 National Diet and Nutrition Survey of pre-school children, dietary habits were assessed, and a relation was observed between the use of carbonated drinks and erosion, especially when consumed at night-time.

It may seem surprising now, from the ethical viewpoint, that a clinical trial was conducted (published in 1957) testing the erosiveness of grapefruit juice, orange juice, and a cola drink, with a control group. The group that consumed the grapefruit juice or the cola drink had the most erosion followed by the orange drink.

## Experimental clinical/animal/in vitro studies

Experimental clinical studies, animal studies, and *in vitro* studies have investigated the erosiveness of various fruit juices and acids. The results appear to confirm that grapefruit juice is amongst the most erosive of fruit juices. Interpretation of the results of many of these studies is difficult, as some authors emphasize the importance of the pH of the drink, while other authors have emphasized the importance of the type of acid (which have different p$K$), and others the 'titratable acidity'. Probably all are important. Animal experiments have shown that phosphoric acid is very erosive at pH 2.5 but much less so at pH 3.3, while lactic acid at pH 4.0 was as destructive as phosphoric acid at pH 2.5. Citric, malic, and tartaric acids are thought to be especially erosive because of their acidic nature and, at higher pH, their ability to chelate calcium. Carbonic acid is thought to be the least erosive acid and carbonated water is not seen as an erosive threat. Fruit-flavoured carbonated waters may pose a threat but information on these is lacking.

Historically, iron tonics have had a very bad reputation for causing dental erosion: their pH was sometimes as low as pH 1.5. Some liquid oral medicines still have a low pH and their erosive potential should be suspected. The recent growth in the use of oral rinses has resulted in some complaints that some of them are erosive, but these suspicions have yet to be clarified.

There is much work being done at present on the effectiveness of adding protective factors (usually calcium based) to drinks to reduce their erosive potential—these important developments will be discussed later in this chapter.

# Who is at risk?

The two most important factors in explaining differences in susceptibility to erosion between individuals are likely to be tooth structure and saliva. Rates of dissolution of teeth vary in laboratory experiments, so that it can be expected that differences in the risk of erosion will vary between individuals. Measuring this *in vivo* is much more difficult and has not yet been attempted. Teeth from people who have lived life-long in fluoridated communities dissolve less readily in acid buffers than teeth from people living in low fluoridated areas. However, there are as yet no reports that water fluoridation confers any protection from erosion, although work on this is in progress.

We are on slightly firmer scientific ground with saliva, since several dental researchers have investigated the relationship between saliva and erosion. All of these authors reported that the unstimulated (resting) saliva flow rate was lower in people with erosion. The importance of both salivary flow rate and diet is illustrated by two studies which have investigated salivary flow and dietary factors: in one study salivary flow was more important than diet, while in the other study it was the other way round.

Since buffering power, and calcium and phosphorus concentrations are directly related to flow rate, it is not surprising that these factors have also been related directly to erosion. A number of diseases (e.g. Sjögren's disease) and drugs (e.g. antidepressants, sedatives, and tranquillizers) severely reduce resting and stimulated salivary flow rates. Some of these drugs, which reduce salivary flow, may also cause nausea and vomiting, making the individual doubly at risk from erosion.

## Case report

Andrea has had asymptomatic gastro-oesophageal reflux for a number of years and as a consequence of sialodectomy to control drooling, has lost salivary gland function. As a result, erosive tooth tissue loss is severe but the patient is asymptomatic (Fig. 4.18).

As far as dietary habits are concerned, four factors are likely to be relevant. The first two are: the time the acid drink or food is in contact with the teeth, and the frequency of consumption. Sipping an acid drink slowly over a long period is likely to be more harmful than drinking it quickly. Three intakes a day will be more harmful than one intake a day.

The third variable is whether the drink or food was taken as part of a meal or separately as a snack. If taken as part of a meal it would seem likely that the acids would be removed or neutralized relatively quickly. The fourth variable is related to the third, as it would also seem likely that acid drinks taken last thing at night may be more damaging because they are not cleared from the mouth so quickly, as salivary flow is very slow during sleep.

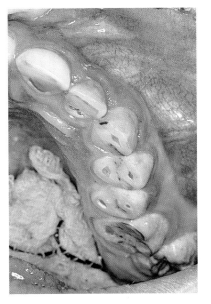

**Figure 4.18** Severe loss of tooth tissue from all permanent teeth as a result of gastro-oesophageal reflux and sialodectomy to control drooling, in this patient with cerebral palsy. The patient is anaesthetized and a throat pack is in place prior to dental care under general anaesthesia.

Box 4.2 **Dietary factors affecting the occurrence of erosion**

The drink
- pH of the drink
- type of acid
- titratable acidity
- protective factors (Ca, P, F)

Method of consumption
- length of time the erosive food or drink is in contact with the teeth (e.g. a can of drink sipped over time)
- frequency of consumption
- other dietary accompaniments (i.e. other food or drinks consumed at the same time)
- timing of foods and drinks (e.g. close to bedtime will be more damaging because of diminished salivary flow)

# How to measure erosion

Our understanding of causes and prevention of dental caries and developmental defects of enamel has been helped considerably by the general use of accepted indices of measurement—the decayed, missing, or filled teeth (DMFT) and the developmental defects of enamel (DDE) indices, respectively. Erosion is more difficult to measure and a useful, easily reproducible index has yet to be established. This is further complicated by the difficulty of differentiating erosion from attrition and abrasion. The most widely used index at present is the 'tooth wear index' (TWI; Table 4.6) proposed by Smith and Knight.

Any index for use in monitoring erosion in patients has to be sufficiently sensitive to record small changes over time. This undoubtedly makes the index less simple to use since deciding between one category and another is sometimes difficult. Another way of monitoring erosion is the use of stone casts obtained from silicone-based impression materials. Unfortunately, because the erosive elements remove microns or more of the whole surface, any landmarks disappear so that visually comparing models, even those made from a silicone-based impression, are unreliable in recording changes over time. Novel techniques for scanning models may become more widespread, once their use has been validated. Clinical photographs are open to the same criticism but, like models, will record the more gross changes. Concurrently in the monitoring process, sequential diet histories from the patient may serve to heighten their awareness of the potential for damage to occur.

The major decisions to be made when examining a surface for erosion are—Is enamel missing? Is dentine exposed? The first is important since it indicates that there may be a problem. From a health promotion point of view, we can then counsel the patient to ensure that the risk is minimized and valuable enamel does not continue to be lost. When dentine is affected, the challenge is greater. Again, we need to identify the cause but also treat if indicated: there may be sensitivity, loss of occlusal vertical dimension, as well as the need to protect the

Table 4.6.
The tooth wear index (TWI)

| Score[a] | Surface | Criterion |
|---|---|---|
| 0 | B/L/Oc/I | No loss of enamel surface characteristics |
| | C | No change of contour |
| 1 | B/L/Oc/I | Loss of enamel surface characteristics |
| | C | Minimal loss of contour |
| 2 | B/L/Oc | Loss of enamel exposing dentine for less than one third of the surface |
| | I | Loss of enamel just exposing dentine |
| | C | A defect less than 1 mm deep |
| 3 | B/L/Oc | Loss of enamel exposing dentine for more than one third of the surface |
| | I | Loss of enamel and substantial loss of dentine, but not exposing pulp or secondary dentine |
| | C | A defect between 1and 2 mm deep |
| 4 | B/L/Oc | Complete loss of enamel, or pulp exposure, or exposure of secondary dentine |
| | I | Pulp exposure or exposure of secondary dentine |
| | C | A defect more than 2 mm deep, or pulp exposure, or exposure of secondary dentine |

[a] In case of doubt the lower score is given.
B = buccal;
L = lingual or palatal;
I = incisal;
Oc = occlusal;
C = cervical.
*Missing* teeth should be scored *M*
*Restored* surfaces should not be scored unless loss of tooth tissue can clearly be seen. Restored surfaces and other unscorable surfaces—e.g. those with extensive caries or fractured incisors should be scored *R*.

surface from further loss. Where anterior teeth are affected because of chipping, flattening of the labial surface, or darkening of the teeth, these aesthetic considerations will need to be addressed as well.

# Prevention of erosion

At present, prevention of erosion is based more on common sense rather than on evidence-based practice. At its most simplistic, removal of the likely causes will reduce risk. That is easier said than done. Dietary habits are subject to many powerful influences, such as advertisements and peer pressure, and are often difficult to change. A glance at Figure 4.4, showing the rise in soft drink consumption, indicates the challenge. Ways of achieving change in the right direction are discussed in Chapter 10.

Table 4.7.
Practical prevention of erosion

Inform patients of types of foods and drinks that have the greatest erosive potential

Limit the intake of acid drinks to mealtimes

Advocate consumption of a neutral food immediately after a meal (e.g milk or cheese)

Advise use of fluoride mouth-rinse or gel for daily use

Encourage the use of carbonate of soda mouth-rinses in cases of recurrent gastric reflux

Where erosion is marked, fluoride toothpaste can be placed in an occlusal guard during the night or during episodes of vomiting

Advise drinking through a straw with the straw well back in the mouth

Practical steps to take in the prevention of erosion are given in Table 4.7.

It would seem logical that the use of fluoride mouth-rinses and the topical application of fluoride varnishes or neutral gels would slow down the progression of erosion as well as reducing symptoms of sensitivity. So far, no clinical trials on these proposals have been conducted. Several rat experiments have shown, though, that the addition of fluoride to acid drinks and the topical application of fluoride to rats' teeth reduces erosion. It would seem reasonable, therefore, to recommend fluoride mouth-rinses and topical fluoride varnishes to lessen the risk of erosion in susceptible people. The mouth-rinse should be of low acid content, manufactured by a reputable oral care company. Brushing immediately after an acid challenge is to be discouraged; although no evidence exists on the time lapse required to render the acid-challenged enamel surface less susceptible to abrasion: it would seem advisable to recommend that at least 20 minutes should elapse before brushing.

Manufacturers of soft drinks have not been insensitive to the criticism that their products erode teeth. Since teeth consist of calcium and phosphorus, it is logical for manufacturers to consider adding these salts to drinks. Calcium phosphate compounds are rather insoluble and calcium affects the taste and pH of a drink. There are, though, calcium compounds which seem to be acceptable additives and are at present marketed in the UK, Germany, and the USA. One of the most promising is calcium–citrate–malate (CCM)—it is soluble and has little impact on taste. Early indications are that this line of research may substantially reduce the erosive potential of drinks and, in 1998, a soft drink sold in the UK received accreditation from the British Dental Association as a non-erosive drink. This is an important milestone and it is hoped that other drink manufacturers will follow this lead.

## Summary

• Although both caries and erosion are caused by acids dissolving tooth mineral, the aetiology, pathology, and clinical distribution of caries and erosion are quite different. Erosion is the surface loss of tooth tissue occurring on surfaces not covered by plaque. Often erosion, abrasion, and attrition combine to cause tooth wear. Tooth wear can be quantified by the tooth wear index (Table 4.6).

- Dental erosion was largely ignored up to the last decade. The decline in dental caries, the great increase in the consumption of soft drinks, the wider availability of fruits and fruit juices, and the obsession of many young women for slimness may have all contributed to the widely accepted belief that the prevalence of dental erosion has increased. Epidemiology of erosion is young and lack of repeated studies prevents firm conclusions on changes in prevalence.

- The three sources of acids are diet, the stomach, and the environment. Common dietary causes are fruit-flavoured and cola-flavoured soft drinks, citrus fruit, fruit juices, and vinegar-based foods. Dietary supplements such as vitamin C tablets and medicines, either as liquid or as acid-containing chewable tablets, have also been implicated.

- Frequency of consumption, duration of consumption, taken alone as a snack instead of with a meal, and taken last thing at night are considered risk factors.

- Other patient-related risk factors include low salivary flow.

- Prevention relies on spotting signs of erosion early and establishing the cause(s) of the erosion. This can be difficult, particularly when some patients are reluctant to admit to vomiting and may be ignorant of regurgitation.

- Reducing any dietary cause is paramount and involves taking a dietary history and giving personal and practical dietary advice.

- The use of fluoride toothpastes, mouth-rinses, and varnishes can be encouraged, although evidence for their effectiveness is limited at present.

- There are strong indications that the manufacturers of soft drinks will be able to make their drinks less erosive.

## Further reading

Rugg-Gunn, A. J. (1993). *Nutrition and dental health*, Chapter 11. Oxford University Press, Oxford.

ten Cate, J. M. and Imfeld, T. (eds) (1996). Etiology, mechanisms and implications of dental erosion. *Eur. J. Oral. Sci.* 104, 149–244.

# 5

# Nutrition and tissues surrounding the teeth

- The gingivae, periodontal tissues and surrounding alveolar bone

- Nutrition and the oral mucosa

- Further reading

# Nutrition and tissues surrounding the teeth

'Lord Anson was Commander-in-Chief of a squadron of ships sent between 1741 and 1744 on an expedition to the South Seas. He sailed from Portsmouth with almost 2000 men in 6 fighting ships and 2 supply ships. Having circled the world they returned to port after 4 years at sea. But of the 2000 men who had left Portsmouth only 200 returned home, most of the rest having died of scurvy.'

D. P. Thomas 1969

This famous voyage of Lord Anson, which was only one of many such voyages with disastrous consequences, was partially instrumental in stimulating Lind's investigations of scurvy. Lind conducted his experiments just 3 years after Anson returned from his voyage around the world and these experiments are described in Box 5.1. Lind probably did not randomly allocate the patients in his study into the six groups he described and, indeed, it was to be another 200 years

Box 5.1

On the 20th May, 1747, I took twelve patients in the scurvy, on board the Salisbury at sea. Their cases were as similar as I could have them. They all in general had putrid gums, the spots and lassitude, with weakness of their knees. They lay together in one place, being a proper apartment for the sick in the forehold; and had one diet common to all. Two of these were ordered each a quart of cyder a-day. Two others took twenty-five gutts of elixir of vitriol three times a-day, upon an empty stomach. Two others took two spoonfuls of vinegar three times a-day, upon an empty stomach; having their gruels and their other food well acidulated with it, as also the gargle for their mouth. Two of the worst patients, with the tendons in the ham rigid, (a symptom none of the rest had), were put under a course of sea-water. Of this they drank half a pint every day, and sometimes more or less as it operated, by way of gentle physic. Two others had each two oranges and one lemon given them every day. These they ate with greediness, at different times upon an empty stomach. They continued but six days under this course, have the quantity that could be spared. The two remaining patients, took the bigness of a nutmeg three times a-day, of an electuary recommended by a hospital surgeon. The consequence was, that the most sudden and visible good effects were perceived from the use of oranges and lemons; one of these who had taken them, being at the end of six days fit for duty. The spots were not indeed at that time quite off his body, nor his gums sound; but without any other medicine, than a gargarism of elixir vitriol, he became quite healthy before we came to Plymouth, which was on the 16th of June. The other was the best recovered of any in his condition; and being now deemed pretty well, was appointed nurse to the rest of the sick.

before a strictly controlled trial was carried out. The beauty of his experiment, though, was that it was a concurrent study under identical conditions comparing various types of therapy commonly used for the treatment of scurvy at that time. Lind declared; 'I shall propose nothing merely dictated from therapy; but shall confirm all by experiment and facts, the surest and most unerring guides'.

Scurvy is a classical nutritional deficiency disease. As a result of Lind's clinical trial, citrus fruits—lime juice in particular—prevented scurvy and British sailors were known as 'limeys' for over a century. Loose teeth and bleeding gums characterize scurvy. Vitamin C is just one of the many nutrients which can affect the supporting tissues of teeth, which is not surprising since tissues surrounding teeth consist of epithelium, connective tissue including collagen and blood vessels, and bone, all of which are known to be affected by deficiencies of various nutrients. It is not only nutrient deficiencies which need to be discussed—the texture of the diet, food allergies, and the possible harmful and protective action of dietary components on the oral mucosa are also relevant.

The tissues surrounding the teeth can be considered under two broad headings. First, the structures which support teeth—the gingivae, periodontal ligament, and the surrounding alveolar bone—and, second, the oral mucosa—principally the epithelium but also the underlying connective tissue.

## The gingivae, periodontal tissues, and surrounding alveolar bone

Periodontal disease is probably man's most prevalent disease—dental caries and periodontal disease vie for this dubious honour. Few escape the destruction of tissues surrounding their teeth. But the severity of periodontal disease varies between areas of the world seemingly quite independently of the prevalence of dental caries. In fact, it was the observations by dental scientists, 50 years ago, who recorded destruction of the supporting tissues around caries-free dentitions, which led to suggestions that nutritional deficiencies were to blame. This view was encouraged by the observation that periodontal disease appeared to be most severe in underdeveloped countries where malnutrition was expected to be most prevalent.

One of the biggest epidemiological studies was conducted by the US Inter-departmental Committee on Nutrition and National Defence in the late 1950s, involving over 22 000 people over the age of 5 years in eight countries (Alaska, Ethiopia, Ecuador, South Vietnam, Chile, Columbia, Thailand, and Lebanon). This study involved an oral examination, a nutritional assessment, and biochemical assays of blood and urine. Over all countries, the amount of dental plaque and age were both highly correlated with severity of periodontal disease. In fact these two factors—plaque quantity and age—explained 90 per cent of the variation in periodontal severity in these populations. The only nutrient found to be significantly related to severity of periodontal disease was serum vitamin A (which is not necessarily a good indicator of vitamin A deficiency) and even this finding was not consistently observed in the different countries. For example, Palestinian refugees in Lebanon with generally acceptable levels of vitamin A showed relatively high levels of disease, while Chilean civilians with acute deficiencies returned average periodontal disease scores. An association between ascorbic acid deficiency and periodontal disease could not be demonstrated in these populations.

A few years later, another important epidemiological study was undertaken under the auspices of the World Health Organization—first in Sri Lanka and then in Norway. A total of over 5000 males and nearly 3000 females aged 13 to over 60 years were examined for both periodontal disease and the presence or absence of vitamins A and B deficiency. As in the above worldwide study, periodontal disease was found to be strongly related to levels of oral hygiene (extent of plaque) and age. Clinical signs of vitamin A deficiency were not associated with severity of periodontal disease, unlike in the extensive studies mentioned above where *serum* vitamin A levels were associated, but inconsistently, with periodontal disease. On the contrary, clinical signs of vitamin B deficiency were associated with higher periodontal disease scores and this association was stronger when the level of oral hygiene was poor.

These Norwegian researchers were impressed by the severity of periodontal disease in Sinhalese and Tamils in Sri Lanka and, on return to Norway, examined 200 Norwegian male service recruits to compare with the data of male Sri Lankan students of the same age. Periodontal disease was indeed more severe in the Sri Lankan sample compared with the Norwegian group, but this could be explained wholly by the higher plaque levels in the Sri Lankan sample (Fig. 5.1). So, from the epidemiological viewpoint, plaque quantity and age seem to be of overriding importance as determinants of periodontal disease.

These limited epidemiological data may not provide the complete picture as both these studies were of cross-sectional design. Three points are relevant. First,

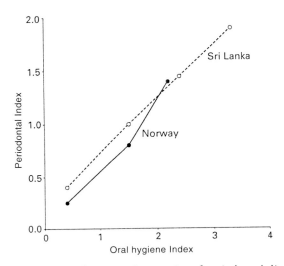

**Figure 5.1** The association between the severity of periodontal disease and oral hygiene observed in 206 Norwegian recruits and in 281 Sri Lankan students aged 19–21 years. Source: Waerhaug (1967).

**Table 5.1.**
Factors concerned with the pathogenesis of periodontal disease which may be influenced by diet and nutrition

Dental plaque (amount and consistency)
Epithelial integrity
Immune response
Collagen formation and repair
Bone formation and repair
Food consistency (fibrous or soft)

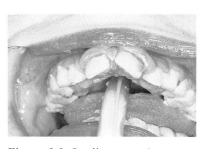

**Figure 5.2** Swollen gums in a patient (under general anaesthesia) who has a vitamin C deficiency. The teeth are also mobile.

it must be remembered that periodontal disease develops very slowly and that any nutritional evaluation is likely to have been limited to a short period and may not reflect lifetime nutritional status. Second, nutritional deficiencies could be strongly related to periodontal disease in a few individuals but these occur so rarely that these relationships are not detected in population surveys. Third, valid methods of estimating nutritional status are difficult to apply in epidemiological studies which are often carried out under difficult field conditions.

Thus, there is still uncertainty about whether malnutrition encourages periodontal destruction, but the important message is that the persistent presence of plaque around the gingival margin is by far the most important cause of periodontal disease.

In spite of the predominant importance of plaque in the aetiology of periodontal disease, much research has been published on the effect of various nutrients on periodontal disease. Results of these are summarized in Table 5.2. It would seem unlikely that deficiencies of vitamins A, B, D, E or calcium have any important influence on periodontal health in man. While most reports have been concerned with vitamin deficiencies, a word of warning about the modern habit of abuse of vitamin supplements: hypervitaminosis A is a serious condition, where gingivae may be swollen with bright red marginal discoloration. Folate (folic acid) is usually classed as a B vitamin and its use in periodontal therapy has been proposed, with some support from evidence from human clinical trials. Folic acid is important in DNA synthesis and tissues with a high cellular turnover rate are most likely to be adversely affected by folic acid deficiency. Cellular turnover rate is especially high in the gingival crevicular epithelium, making this tissue especially vulnerable, reducing the ability of this epithelial layer to function as a barrier to bacterial insults.

A number of trials have reported beneficial results from both systemic and topical administration of folate. In one such trial, patients attending a periodontal clinic rinsed twice daily with 5 ml of a mouth-rinse containing 5 mg folate and had a significant decrease in gingivitis after 4 weeks compared with a control group who rinsed with a placebo.

During pregnancy, the gingival tissues can exhibit an exaggerated vascular response to plaque and it has been suggested that this reaction could be due to 'end tissue deficiency' of folic acid. To test this hypothesis, 30 pregnant women were randomly allocated to three groups. Group A received a placebo mouth-rinse and a placebo tablet, group B a placebo mouth rinse and one folic acid tablet daily, group C a folic acid mouth rinse and a placebo tablet. Supplementation lasted for 14 days during months 4 and 8 of pregnancy. The folate mouth-rinse but not the folate tablets produced a significant improvement in gingival health. Similar results were obtained testing supplementation for 28 days during the eighth month only—a significant improvement in gingival health for the group using the folate mouth-rinse was observed. These results give credence to the end tissue deficiency hypothesis.

Vitamin C is one nutrient which is clearly related to periodontal disease in some patients. Deficiency of vitamin C leads to scurvy, a recognized sign and symptom of which is swollen, bleeding gums (Fig 5.2), which is both prevented

Table 5.2.
Nutrient deficiencies and periodontal disease

| Nutrient | Action of nutrient | Demonstrated in animal experiments | Observation in man | Therapeutic use in man |
|---|---|---|---|---|
| Vitamin A | Required for maintenance of epithelial tissue | Marginal gingivitis, gingival bone hypoplasia, pocket formation, alveolar resorption | Some epidemiological surveys have linked deficiency to increased periodontal disease | No benefit demonstrated |
| Vitamin B | Many B vitamins are coenzymes concerned with intracellular metabolism, especially carbohydrate metabolism | Gingival inflammation, epithelial necrosis, resorption of alveolar bone | Recorded in one epidemiological study | No studies reported |
| Folic acid | Concerned with DNA synthesis and maturation of red blood cells | | No reports, but see therapeutic use | Reduction of gingivitis following either systemic or topical use (as mouth rinse); topical use gives the greater effect |
| Vitamin C | Key role in collagen synthesis | Extensive evidence of effect on periodontal tissues | Clearly recorded. One of the classical signs of scurvy | Results of many trials have been mixed—some positive, some negative. Results of trials of 'mega-doses' have been negative |
| Vitamin D | Promotes absorption and retention of calcium | Much evidence: osteoporosis in alveolar bone; overdosing can lead to osteosclerosis | No reports | No studies reported |
| Vitamin E | Antioxidant; maintains cell membranes | No effect on periodontal tissues | No reports | One trial suggests reduction in gingivitis after supplementation |
| Calcium and phosphorus | Essential for bone formation and maintenance; intimately involved with vitamin D | Osteoporosis of alveolar bone; low Ca:P ratio especially damaging | No reports | Mixed results from a few clinical trials of Ca supplementation |
| Fluoride | Affinity for calcified tissues | Fluorides reduce osteoporosis | Some evidence that periodontal disease is less in areas with adequate F in water | Mainly for prevention of dental caries. Some F compounds (e.g. $SnF_2$) effective |
| Energy and protein | Deficiency leads to failure to thrive; starvation; suppression of immune response | Degradation of connective tissue of gingivae and periodontal ligament; osteoporosis of alveolar bone | No changes observed despite 24% weight loss; neutropenia associated with severe periodontal disease | Short trials have suggested that protein supplementation decreases gingival inflammation and sulcus depth |
| Carbohydrates | Main source of energy. Intraorally, sugars are converted to acids by plaque bacteria | Dietary sugars have a contributing role in progressive periodontal disease | Sugar restriction results in less plaque, but effect on gingivitis is minimal | Short trials show reduced plaque and gingival bleeding with reduced sugar intake |

Based on: McLaren D S (1992) Diet related disorders

and cured by adequate intake of vitamin C. Vitamin C has many metabolic functions but the most important is its key role in collagen synthesis. This is relevant not only to the maintenance of tissues, such as the periodontal ligament (which consists principally of collagen fibres), but also the formation of bone matrix and maintenance of the integrity of blood vessel walls.

Scurvy is uncommon and usually confined to solo elderly patients consuming 'bread and tea' diets (with or without alcohol); occasionally it is seen in infants fed on heat-treated cow's milk. The signs and symptoms of scurvy have been reported in five male prisoners who were given vitamin C deficient diets for up to 97 days. Haemorrhagic lesions were seen in the skin as early as day 29, but it was not until several weeks later that bleeding gums were noticed. Other later symptoms included joint pains and a reduction in salivary flow. The gingivae in scurvy are swollen and bluish-red in colour and prone to spontaneous bleeding. The teeth become loose due to breakdown of the periodontium and there is a widening of the periodontal ligament space which can be seen on radiographs.

Most epidemiological studies have failed to demonstrate a relationship between ascorbic acid intake and periodontal disease. Intake of ascorbic acid in amounts larger than those recommended by dietary standards does not seem to be associated with better periodontal health. This latter finding is important since some dentists have recommended mega-doses (1 g per day) of vitamin C as part of therapy for periodontal disease. The results of clinical trials do not support the use of mega-doses of vitamin C in normal subjects for this purpose. If you were to consider the use of large doses of vitamins or other nutrients, it would be sensible to seek professional dietetic advice.

## Fluoride

The caries-preventive effect of fluoride was shown clearly in Chapter 4. In contrast, there is much less information on the effect of fluoride on gingivitis and periodontitis and most of this information comes from epidemiological studies of dental health of children and adults living in areas receiving different fluoride levels in their public water supplies.

Studies of the level of gingivitis in children yield mixed results with some studies reporting less gingivitis in children living in areas receiving near optimum fluoride levels (about 1 mg F/l) than in children living in areas with low fluoride levels, while other studies reported no difference in gingivitis scores between high and low fluoride areas. No studies have been reported in which gingivitis was more severe in the fluoride compared with the non-fluoride community.

There have been a few epidemiological surveys of periodontal disease in adults who have been lifelong residents in areas receiving optimum or low levels of fluoride in their public water supplies. In a fairly large study of 18–70 year olds living in Aurora (1.2 mg F/l) and Rockford, USA (0.1 mg F/l), more periodontal destruction was observed in each age group in lifelong residents of Rockford. Since the standard of oral cleanliness was the same in both populations, the authors suggested that the reduced severity of periodontal disease was either an indirect effect of the lower prevalence of dental caries in Aurora or a direct effect of fluoride on alveolar bone resorption.

## Carbohydrates

There have been several investigations in both animals and human subjects of the effect of carbohydrate restriction or addition on the quantity and quality of plaque formed and the development of gingivitis. Most of the studies have investigated sugars rather than starches, or carbohydrate as a whole. Several studies, usually lasting a few weeks, have shown that supplementing the diet with sugars increases the quantity of plaque and gingival bleeding. Conversely, restriction of dietary sugar over 2 years resulted in reduced plaque formation and a weak trend towards less gingivitis.

## Fibre and food consistency

Apples have often been seen as a symbol of dental health. Fruit and fibrous foods have been discussed briefly in Chapter 4 in relation to dental caries, and their effect on periodontal health will now be summarized. Fibrous foods, and apples in particular, have often been viewed as nature's toothbrush—cleaning away plaque which is so important in periodontal disease. In a long review of this subject, 50 years ago and which listed 103 references, it was concluded that 'the weight of existing evidence strongly favours the conclusion that the physical character of the diet bares significant relations to the health of periodontal tissues'. There seem to be three recurring themes—that fibrous foods

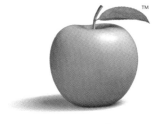

Denplan

**Figure 5.3** An apple and oral health have always been synonymous. Reproduced with permission of Denplan.

- 'exercise the gums';
- 'keratinize the gingivae'; and
- 'clean the teeth'.

Evidence does not support all these statements. While several studies have shown that animals eating soft diets develop more plaque and gingivitis than animals fed on a fibrous diet, this has not been demonstrated in humans except under extreme circumstances. Several workers have investigated the effect of chewing apples or carrots daily on gingival health and the results were with one exception negative. The most likely explanation for this lack of effect in humans is the difference in shape of human teeth compared with, for example, the shape of a dog's teeth. While fibrous foods may remove plaque from exposed surfaces of teeth, the area around the gingival margin (the important area for the initiation of periodontal disease) seems to be little affected by fibrous foods. No evidence exists showing that chewing fibrous foods increases gingival keratinization in humans or that this reduces or protects against gingivitis. Chewing increases salivary flow and this speeds up clearance of food residue from the mouth but, although this is likely to aid dental caries prevention, it has not been shown to benefit gingival health. On the favourable side, fibrous foods tend to be 'healthy foods' and low in non-milk extrinsic sugars and, for this reason, they are likely to benefit oral health.

Chewing seems to have a beneficial effect on the periodontal membranes and alveolar bone—by production of thicker and well-developed fibre bundles in the periodontal membrane and well-structured non-atrophic bone—but this evidence was collected over 50 years ago and there seem to be little recent data. So, in summary, it would appear that in humans, fibrous foods

- do not remove plaque from areas adjacent to gingival tissues;
- do not increase keratinization of the gingival epithelium;
- may help to maintain the supporting tissues of teeth (bone and periodontal ligament);
- increase clearance of foods from the mouth by increasing salivary flow, but this would appear to be of little relevance to periodontal disease;
- are generally low in non-milk extrinsic sugars and are therefore a good substitute for foods high in non-milk extrinsic sugars which cause dental caries and increase plaque growth.

But they are not a substitute for careful tooth-brushing in modern societies.

## Summary

The periodontal tissues are composed of epithelium, collagen fibres, blood vessels, other connective tissue elements, cementum, and bone. It would be very surprising if nutritional deficiencies did not adversely effect these tissues. There is strong evidence of adverse effects from experiments on rats, guinea pigs, and dogs, but there is much less evidence in humans. Only in the case of scurvy (ascorbic acid deficiency) are the periodontal tissues primarily affected. Overall, periodontal tissues will benefit when nutrition is adequate, but dietary supplementation of nutrients above what is commonly accepted as adequate levels does not seem to improve periodontal health further. Inadequate levels of folate appear to exist in gingival tissues in defined groups of people and delivery of folate to these tissues locally in the mouth (for example in a mouth-rinse) can be beneficial. By far the most important way of maintaining periodontal health in humans is regular, thorough, physical removal of dental plaque with a satisfactory toothbrush.

# Nutrition and the oral mucosa

'The mouth is the mirror of the body' is an old saying and has much truth. A look at the tongue was often a regular part of a doctor's examination of his patient. While the tongue is usually pink and rough from the presence of filiform and fungiform papillae, a whitish tongue (where the tongue is covered with a layer very similar to dental plaque) indicated that the patient was 'under the weather'. A red or ulcerated tongue, or a tongue covered in a thick white layer would indicate something more serious. Although the tongue is the most revealing part of 'the mirror', the lips, especially the corners (or commissures) of the lips and the rest of the oral mucosa can also be affected. Nutrition is, of course, only one of the many factors affecting the appearance of the oral mucosa. This part of the chapter will be divided into three sections—a consideration of nutritional deficiency diseases, food allergies, and oral cancer.

## Nutritional deficiencies

Watch out for the red painful tongue and angular stomatitis! Table 5.3 gives more detailed information. As can be seen, it is the water-soluble B vitamins

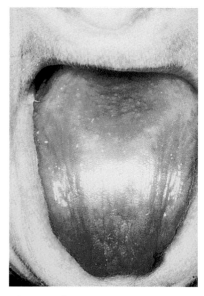

**Figure 5.4** The red, smooth tongue of a patient deficient in B vitamins. Reproduced with permission of Dr A Nolan.

which indicate their nutritional deficiency in the oral tissues. Iron deficiency is sometimes intimately involved with some B vitamin deficiencies and can also be suspected from the appearance of the mouth. For many of these vitamin B deficiencies, the tongue is smooth through loss of filiform or fungiform papillae (or often both types)—a red and painful tongue. While niacin deficiency is characterized by a scarlet tongue, riboflavin and biotin deficiencies are characterized by magenta-coloured tongues. If anaemia is severe, the tongue will be pale rather than red. Atrophy of the edges of the tongue in vitamin $B_{12}$ deficiency is said to mirror the atrophy of the gastric lining in these patients.

Angular stomatitis is inflammation and cracking of the corners or commissures of the lips; it is also called angular cheilitis. It is seen commonly in deficiencies of iron, as well as deficiencies of vitamins $B_{12}$ and $B_2$. Generalized inflammation of the lips (cheilosis) is also seen in vitamin $B_2$ deficiency.

Aphthous ulcers are very painful, often discreet ulcers and frequently in the oral mucosal sulci. Their aetiology is poorly understood, but it would appear that deficiency of folate and/or iron may be initiating factors.

How common are these deficiency diseases of the oral mucosa? In the UK, probably not common, but they are still endemic in several areas of the developing world. The most common in the UK is likely to be recurrent aphthous

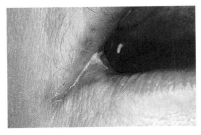

**Figure 5.5** Angular cheilitis as a consequence of deficiencies of iron and vitamins $B_2$ and $B_{12}$. Reproduced with permission of Dr A Nolan.

## Table 5.3.
## Nutrient deficiencies and the oral mucosa

| Nutrient | Main general clinical features | Tongue | Lips and/or the oral mucosa |
|---|---|---|---|
| Vitamin $B_{12}$ (cobalamin) | Abnormalities of bone marrow, small intestine and nervous system Occasionally, hyperpigmentation of skin | Smooth (filiform papillae atrophy) Red (or pale if anaemia is marked) and sore Atrophy of edges | Angular stomatitis ? Aphthous ulceration |
| Folate | Megaloblastic anaemia Occasionally, hyperpigmented skin | Smooth (filiform papillae atrophy) Red (or pale if anaemia is marked) and painful | ? Aphthous ulceration |
| Vitamin $B_6$ (pyridoxine) | Peripheral neuropathy | Red and swollen (glossitis) | Inflamed lips |
| Niacin | Disease (pellagra) of the '3 D's— dermatitis, diarrhoea, dementia | Smooth (filiform papillae atrophy) Scarlet Extremely painful | Nil |
| Vitamin $B_2$ (riboflavin) | Rather unspecific—rash around nose and oral signs | Magenta | Angular stomatitis Cheilosis |
| Biotin | Fatigue, nausea, muscle pains, scaly skin | Magenta; swollen and painful | Red and sore oral mucosa |
| Iron | Anaemia Koilonychia (spoon-shaped nails) Dysplasia | Smooth (filiform papillae atrophy) Painful, may be pale | Angular stomatitis ? Aphthous ulceration |

Based on: McLaren, D S (1992) Diet related disorders.

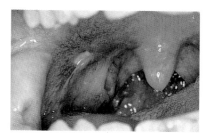

**Figure 5.6** An aphthous ulcer near the pillar of the fauces.

**Investigation of recurrent aphthous ulceration (RAS)**

FBC—looking for neutropenia

Serum ferritin—as this is in equilibrium with ferritin stores in the body

Red cell folate

Serum vitamin $B_{12}$

**Investigations for angular cheilitis**

Serum ferritin

Vitamin $B_{12}$

Blood glucose

Swabs: eyes, nostrils, intraoral, and dentures

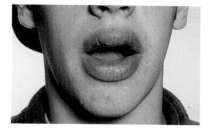

**Figure 5.7** Swelling of the lips in a patient with orofacial granulomatosis. Reproduced with permission of Dr A Nolan.

stomatitis (RAS) and sideropenia. Falling concentration of haemoglobin is a sign of anaemia; sideropenia precedes anaemia and may be evident in the mouth long before anaemia. Iron, vitamin $B_{12}$, and folate deficiency is present in about 20 per cent of people with recurrent aphthous ulceration in developed countries. Establishing whether nutritional deficiency is associated with aphthous ulceration requires laboratory investigations. These include a full blood count, serum ferritin, vitamin $B_{12}$, and red cell folate levels; nutritional supplementation will depend on the findings. A full blood count on its own is not a good indicator of ferritin, vitamin $B_{12}$ or folate deficiency as mean corpuscular volume (MCV) is not a sensitive method of detecting macrocytic/microcytic anaemias. There is a 60 per cent resolution of signs and symptoms if patients are given the appropriate supplementation.

### Noma

Noma is a disease of the oral region strongly linked to malnutrition: it is also known as cancrum oris or orofacial gangrene. It most commonly occurs in Africa, where the prevalence is one to seven per 1000 population. It tends to occur in children aged 3–16 years and genders are equally affected. The perioral flesh is the first to be destroyed. If untreated, mortality is very high. The cause of noma has yet to be determined but it is very strongly linked to malnutrition, with deficiencies of zinc and vitamins A and C being suggested. Acute ulcerative gingivitis may be a precursor; it may be linked to foot-rot in animals, as close proximity to domestic animals appears to be a risk factor. Prevention will rely on the prevention of severe malnutrition.

## Food allergies

Although food allergy is a common term, 'food intolerance' or 'food sensitivity' are to be preferred. Allergy is different from intolerance as only the former provokes an antibody response. 'Food adversion' usually refers to psychological avoidance of foods. All these come under the broad umbrella of 'adverse reactions to foods'. Foods are only one of the many causes of sensitivities—pollen and penicillin come to mind as two non-food examples. The protein component of foods is usually responsible. Sensitivity reactions can be immediate and life threatening or delayed, and it is common to classify these reactions as type I (fast) to IV (slow).

It is difficult to estimate the prevalence of food intolerances. A questionnaire survey of adults in the UK suggested that 20 per cent of the population had intolerance to one or more foods. However, supervised challenge tests reduced the prevalence of actual sensitivity to below 2 per cent. Many people blame food additives for adverse reactions but, according to the Ministry of Agriculture, Fisheries and Food, sensitivity reactions to food additives probably affect only one in 10 000 people. Small children are more likely to react to certain foods, probably because of immaturity of their gut. Perhaps one in ten young children in the UK are affected in this way but eight out of ten of these grow out of it. This especially applies to milk sensitivity.

As food is taken in through the mouth, it is not surprising that signs and symptoms of adverse reactions to foods and drinks sometimes affect the lips, mouth, throat, and skin close to the mouth (Table 5.4). Symptoms of these oral effects are usually swelling, a rash, and/or itching. Colouring and preservatives appear to be the most likely to cause perioral symptoms (Table 5.5). It is worth noting that these clinical effects are not due to contact allergy alone but due also to a primed T-cell reaction. The possibility of food sensitivity should be borne in mind when giving dietary advice to patients. This especially applies to nuts and milk. Dietary advice is considered in detail in Chapter 10.

Sometimes the food responsible can be identified fairly easily but, on the whole, investigation of food sensitivity is a difficult task and should be left to experienced clinicians. Isolation of the dietary item responsible usually involves a very careful history but, more importantly, by exclusion diets and food challenge tests. Included as part of these would be specific testing, because type IV reactions can occur after 3–7 days post-contact; identification from a history is almost impossible.

### Table 5.4.
### Signs and symptoms associated with food allergy

| | |
|---|---|
| Oral | Swollen lips, itching, swelling of the mouth and throat |
| Skin | Urticaria (rash), itching, eczema (especially atophic eczema), redness |
| Gastrointestinal | Abdominal pain, abdominal distension, vomiting, diarrhoea |
| Respiratory | Runny nose, sneezing, wheezing, asthma |
| Neurological | Irritability, restlessness, hyperactivity, migraine |
| Other | Anaphylaxis |

Based on: McLaren D S (1992) Diet related disorders

### Table 5.5.
### Foods commonly associated with sensitivity reactions

| | |
|---|---|
| Oral | Colourings (e.g. tartrazine), preservatives (e.g. benzoate) |
| Skin | Egg, cow's milk, wheat, colourings, perservatives |
| Gastrointestinal | Egg, cow's milk, nuts, seafood, some fruits |
| Respiratory | Egg, nuts, fish, chocolate, colourings, preservatives |
| Migraine | Cheese, tomatoes, chocolate, cow's milk, egg, orange |
| Angio-oedema and anaphylaxis | Peanuts, egg, fish, cow's milk |

Based on: McLaren D S (1992) Diet related disorders

## A nutty problem for nursing mothers

A CORRESPONDENT to *The Times* was worried as to why allergy to peanuts has only recently become an important health issue. In fact peanut allergy has been recognised for many years but it is now a growing problem, with one person in 200 being allergic to peanuts.

Peanut butter, once so beloved by nanny in the nursery and a well-remembered part of the wartime diet, is now thought to be one of the ways in which children are sensitised to it. Peanut-rich foods, whether taken by a pregnant woman or lactating mother, may also sensitise the foetus or newborn infant. Professor John Warner of Southampton University associates maternal consumption of peanuts with the increasing prevalence of the allergy and its earlier onset. Research suggests that antigens from the peanut-eating mother cross the placenta barrier, and other studies have shown that the unborn baby can become allergic to peanuts as a result of swallowing the amniotic fluid of a woman who may, for instance, have eaten too many peanuts with her evening drink.

The Department of Health suggests that peanuts are not an essential part of anyone's diet and should be avoided by women with a family history of allergies. Children under three with a similar family history should not have peanut products.

*Times 9.7.98*

**Figure 5.8** Much publicity has centred recently around nut allergies, including the likelihood of transfer by the mother to her breastfed baby, as indicated in this headline.

## Oral cancer

The World Health Organization estimated that in 1996 there were over ten million new cases of cancer and that over seven million people died from cancer. The figures for men and women are given separately in Table 5.6. It can be seen that cancers of the mouth and pharynx were the fifth most common cancers in men and the sixth most common in women. For both genders combined, cancer of the mouth and pharynx ranks fifth, with an estimated 575 000 new cases, accounting for 5.6 per cent of all new cases in 1996. Survival rates are better for oral cancer than for some other cancers, so that cancer of the mouth and pharynx ranks sixth as the cause of cancer deaths in men and women. All the cancers listed in Table 5.6 are believed to be related to diet, including lung cancer, where of course cigarette smoking is established as a major risk factor.

Table 5.6.
### Estimated numbers of new cases and deaths from cancer worldwide—1996

| Cancer site | New cases (thousands) | Percentage of total | Deaths (thousands) | Percentage of total |
|---|---|---|---|---|
| **Men** | | | | |
| Lung | 988 | 18.6 | 878 | 22.4 |
| Stomach | 634 | 11.9 | 518 | 13.2 |
| Colon, rectum | 445 | 8.4 | 257 | 6.6 |
| Prostate | 400 | 7.5 | 204 | 5.2 |
| Mouth and pharynx | 384 | 7.2 | 237 | 6.1 |
| Liver | 374 | 7.1 | 370 | 9.4 |
| Oesophagus | 320 | 6.1 | 305 | 7.8 |
| Bladder | 236 | 4.4 | 107 | 2.7 |
| Other | 1531 | 28.8 | 1043 | 26.6 |
| Total | 5312 | 100.0 | 3919 | 100.0 |
| **Women** | | | | |
| Breast | 910 | 18.2 | 390 | 12.2 |
| Cervix | 524 | 10.5 | 241 | 7.6 |
| Colon, rectum | 431 | 8.6 | 253 | 7.9 |
| Stomach | 379 | 7.6 | 317 | 9.9 |
| Lung | 333 | 6.7 | 282 | 8.8 |
| Mouth and pharynx | 192 | 3.8 | 129 | 4.1 |
| Ovary | 191 | 3.8 | 125 | 3.9 |
| Endometrium | 172 | 3.4 | 68 | 2.1 |
| Other | 1874 | 37.4 | 1387 | 43.5 |
| Total | 5006 | 100.0 | 3192 | 100.0 |

World Cancer Research Fund, American Institute for Cancer Research.

The relative importance of various cancers varies throughout the world depending on the relative strength of various risk and protective factors. In Bombay, for example, cancers of the mouth and pharynx account for 18 per cent of all male cancers followed by cancers of the lung, oesophagus, and larynx. The rates of cancers for many sites have changed, in many cases remarkably in recent decades. Rates for most of the common cancers have increased, with the exception of stomach cancer which has decreased. Between 1996 and 2020 the total number of cases of cancer in the developing world is expected to double and in the developed world to increase by 40 per cent.

There have been various estimates of the relative importance that diet plays in the pathogenesis of cancer. In 1981, Doll and Peto estimated that at least one third of human cancers could be related directly to some dietary component—in the European community, this would mean that some half a million new cases of cancer each year would have a major dietary basis. Furthermore, it seems plausible that nutrition plays a permissive role in enhancing the development of many other cancers, so that up to 80 per cent of all cancers may have a link with nutrition. Thus, as this represents about one million new cases of cancer per year in the EC, changes in nutritional intake could induce major changes in cancer rates, and it is not surprising that this is an area of intense research and health promotion.

## Mouth and pharynx

The incidence of mouth and pharyngeal cancers is twice as common in the developing world where nearly 80 per cent of cases occur. In developed countries, recent trends show an increase in incidence and mortality—for example, in Europe, Japan, and Australia. Cancers of the mouth and pharynx include those of the tongue, gums, floor of the mouth, and other parts of the mouth and pharynx. Cancers of the lip (predominantly influenced by sunlight and smoking) and of the salivary glands are outside this classification.

By far the most important dietary influence on the occurrence of oral cancer is alcohol. The evidence is extensive and consistent. For example, reports of six retrospective and five prospective cohort studies yielded relative risks of between 1.3 and 8.6. Nineteen case–control studies gave odds ratios of between 1.3 and 7.2 (i.e. these people were 1.3 to 7.2 times more likely to have oral cancer compared with others who did not practice the habit(s) of the affected people). For any given level of alcohol intake, there is no clear difference in risk associated with specific types of alcoholic drinks. Although an early study in the USA found the highest relative risk in whisky drinkers, subsequent studies have reported similar risks of cancer of the mouth and pharynx among drinkers of different types of drink—wines, beers, whisky, and mixed drinks.

It is very likely that there are synergistic interactions between alcohol consumption and tobacco use: individuals with high exposure to both alcohol and tobacco have a relative risk of 15.6 compared with those who neither smoke nor drink alcohol.

In common with other upper aero-digestive cancers, tobacco and alcohol probably act as sources of direct-acting agents that damage DNA. There is a multitude of carcinogens in tobacco—both chewed and smoked (Fig. 5.11)—and the first metabolic products of alcohol acetaldehyde can adduct to DNA.

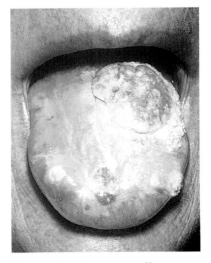

**Figure 5.9** Oral cancer affecting the ventral surface of the tongue. Reproduced with permission of Dr A Nolan.

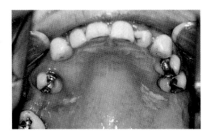

**Figure 5.10** White, keratotic lesions on the hard palate of this patient who drinks and smokes heavily.

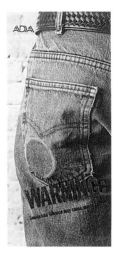

**Figure 5.11** A leaflet from North America promoting the use of smokeless tobacco.

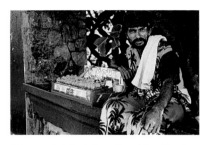

**Figure 5.12** A betel-quid seller in Sri Lanka with a tray containing ready prepared betel-quid.

Box 5.3

---

### Odds ratio (OR)

Odds are the ratio of the probability that something will occur to the probability that something will not occur. This can be calculated separately for those people who have a particular factor (e.g. who smoke) and for those who do not have a particular factor (e.g. do not smoke). The ratio of these is the odds ratio. The odds ratio indicates the odds in favour of having the disease with the factor present compared with having the factor absent.

### Relative risk (RR)

Relative risk is the ratio of the incidence rate for persons exposed to a factor to the incidence rate for those not exposed.

Both OR and RR indicate the increased risk of having a particular factor or undertaking a particular activity.

---

Further, alcohol can facilitate the entry of tobacco carcinogens into cells as a result of its solvent properties. Finally, both alcohol and tobacco damage cells, thus inducing a compensatory hyper-proliferation that increases the likelihood of persistence of unrepaired DNA damage across generations of cells.

Betel-quid chewing has long been linked to oral cancer—studies as long ago as 1933 suggested this. Although there are several and varied ingredients of the betel-quid, only tobacco has been clearly related to oral cancer.

Of all the other dietary constituents, vegetables and fruit have consistently been associated with decreased risk of cancer of the mouth and pharynx. Thirteen out of 15 case–control studies reported statistically significant protective associations for at least one vegetable and/or fruit category, with odds ratios varying from 0.2 to 0.6.

Protective associations for vegetable and fruit consumption have remained significant after adjustment for smoking (or other forms of tobacco consumption such as chewing) and high alcohol consumption. Typically, the risk of cancer of the mouth and pharynx is halved in those who eat fruit/vegetables daily versus less than daily consumption. The evidence is most consistent for carrots, citrus fruits, and green vegetables. Interventional studies on hamsters have shown a 60 per cent reduction in tumour load in the buccal pouch when pretreated with 'leminoids'.

There is no protective association with consumption of pulses, grains, minerals, and vitamins, other than for vitamin C where five case–control studies have consistently reported odds ratios of 0.3 to 0.6. Some other studies also point to the value of vitamins A and E. Vitamins A, C, and E are thought to scavenge potentially mutagenic free radicals from damaged cells.

Data available provide no evidence that coffee or tea consumption increases risk of oral cancer. However, maté is commonly drunk as tea in some parts of South America and would appear to be a risk factor for oral cancer—regular drinkers of maté have approximately a two-fold increase in risk. This may be a

Table 5.7.

Strength of evidence relating food and nutrition to cancer of the mouth and pharynx

| Evidence | Decreases risk | Increases risk |
|---|---|---|
| Convincing | Vegetables and fruits | Alcohol |
| Possible | Vitamin C | Maté[a] |

[a] See text on pp. 92–93.
World Cancer Research Fund, American Institute for Cancer Research.

consequence of the high temperature at which this beverage is usually consumed. There is no other evidence that hot drinks increase risk of oral and pharyngeal carcinoma.

Oral cancer is largely a preventable disease. The role of tobacco as the overwhelming cause of lung cancer, now the most common cancer globally, is well known. However, between 30 and 40 per cent of cancer incidence worldwide is preventable by more healthy eating, weight control, and exercise. It has been estimated that almost 87 per cent of the incidence of cancer of the mouth and pharynx can potentially be reduced by not smoking, reducing alcohol drinking, and increasing consumption of vegetables and fruits. Excluding the non-dietary risk factor of smoking, a diet high in a variety of vegetables and fruits and avoidance of alcohol may prevent between 33 and 50 per cent of cases of cancer of the mouth and pharynx.

# Further reading

Department of Health (1998). *Nutritional aspects of the development of cancer*. Report on health and social subjects, 48. Department of Health, London.

Ferguson, M. M. (1990). Nutritional disorders. In *Oral manifestations of systemic disease* (2nd edn) (ed. M. Jones and D. Mason). Baillière Tindall, London.

McLaren, D. S. (1992). *A colour atlas and text of diet-related disorders* (2nd edn). Wolfe Publishing, London.

Rugg-Gunn, A. J. (1993). *Nutrition and dental health*, Chapter 12. Oxford University Press, Oxford.

Seymour, R. A. and Heasman, P. A. (1992). *Drugs, diseases and the periodontium*. Oxford University Press, Oxford.

WCRF (1997). *Food, nutrition and the prevention of cancer; a global perspective*. World Cancer Research Fund, American Institute for Cancer Research, Washington DC.

WHO (1998). *Noma today; a public health problem? Report of an expert consultation*. WHO/MMC/NOMA/98.1. World Health Organization, Geneva.

**6**

# The value of teeth in nutrition

# The value of teeth in nutrition

## Introduction

In most animals teeth are essential for survival. They are a necessary tool for preparing food for ingestion and a weapon for defence or attack. The loss of teeth leads to an inability of the animal to defend itself and to catch and prepare food. In many animals, once food is taken inside the mouth it has to be chopped or ground before being swallowed to ensure satisfactory digestion. Over the millennia, the human race has depended less and less on teeth for survival. Modern food preparation involving cutting, grinding and cooking has resulted in soft diets which can be eaten easily by people with poor dental health. It would be wrong to say that teeth are totally unimportant for consuming a modern diet, but their role in ensuring an adequate nutrition is very much reduced. Our intelligence and skill have meant that we are able to prepare food so that it is enjoyable to eat and easily digested. Since teeth in modern societies have lost the major part of their most important function—namely food preparation—it has been said that 'the dentition is in a state of hypofunction'. Modern humans use only a fraction of their potential chewing force. Conversely, we are very concerned with appearance and communication and, in most human societies now, by far the most important role for teeth is enhancing appearance. Facial appearance is tremendously important in determining an individual's integration into society (Fig. 6.3).

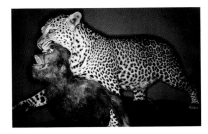

**Figure 6.1** Animals are totally reliant on an intact dentition for survival.

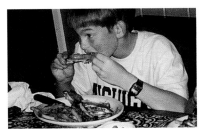

**Figure 6.2** Teeth are of value in tearing meat in many humans as well as animals.

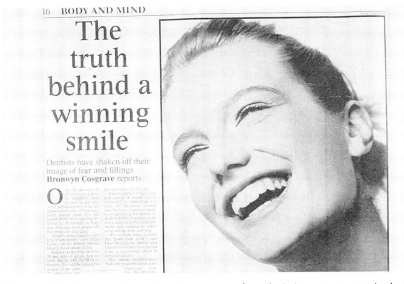

**Figure 6.3** An attractive smile, showing good teeth, is important, particularly in society today.

If our teeth are in a state of hypofunction, are they required at all for adequate or optimal nutrition? It is technically possible to produce complete diets in liquid form. There are two counter arguments: first, a lack of teeth is socially unacceptable to the majority of people and, second, liquid diets are usually (not always) poor in energy—an attribute taken advantage of by purveyors of slimming foods.

Before we consider whether a poor dentition can adversely affect nutrition, it is important to be clear that good nutrition matters. Some points are worth mentioning.

- The increasing height of our population is an indication of better nutrition, particularly with regard to energy and protein intake. On the other hand, obesity in children is increasing so that eating the right foods and exercising are important.

- It is now over 10 years since it became clear that nutrition *in utero* influences the occurrence of disease (e.g. cardiovascular disease) in adulthood. It is well known that excessive consumption of dietary fats is an important risk factor for cardiovascular disease and excessive consumption of sugars the cause of dental caries and probably a risk factor for diabetes.

- In the previous chapter, the ability of the diet to cause and prevent cancer—in almost all systems of the body—was strongly emphasized. About one third of all cancers are preventable by feasible changes in diet.

More specific dietary advice for children and adults is covered in the next two chapters, but suffice to conclude that nutrition is a very important determinant of health and disease. This chapter examines the importance of the quality of the dentition in this relationship.

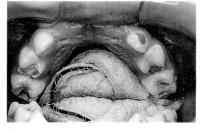

**Figure 6.4** Rampant dental caries in a child from a disadvantaged home background, awaiting general anaesthesia for extractions.

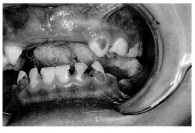

**Figure 6.5** The anterior view of the child in Fig. 6.4.

## Case report

Keith was brought to the attention of the dentist by his health visitor and social worker. He and his sister were looked after some of the time by parents who were both alcoholics; the remainder of the time they were cared for by grandparents. The parents refused to bring the child to the dentist, so a home visit was made. Home circumstances were very poor, as reflected in the child's failure to thrive and the need to have a dental clearance (Figs 6.4 and 6.5), having already had one general anaesthetic for extractions in the previous year.

There is concern that young children having general anaesthesia for dental extractions are lighter in body weight compared with the rest of the child population (Fig. 6.6). Why is this? We might conclude that the child's impaired dentition—perhaps painful teeth or missing teeth—cause undernutrition, on the other hand it could be that the poor diet came first resulting in both carious teeth and undernutrition. It is difficult from cross-sectional studies such as that presented in Fig. 6.6 to conclude which explanation is correct. Nevertheless, it is right to be concerned about the possibility that dental impairment causes undernutrition in children: we need to be aware of this possibility and give dietary

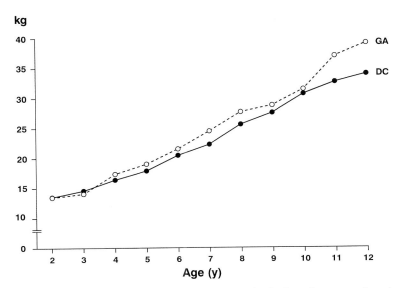

**Figure 6.6** The body weights of 1105 children who had teeth extracted under a general anaesthetic (GA) were lower than those of 527 children who had dental care (DC) and no extractions. Based on: Miller *et al.* (1982).

advice to parents of such children as appropriate. This will be discussed further in Chapters 7 and 10.

Elderly people who have few of their own teeth left, do find eating difficult. The first national survey of nutrition in the elderly in Britain carried out in 1967–8 fortunately included a dental examination. The elderly people who had insufficient mastication (as judged by observation) had a lower energy intake, a lower body mass index (a measure of obesity), and lower skin-fold thickness than those judged to have efficient mastication. The most recent national Diet and Nutrition Survey of people over 65 years of age also confirms that the edentulous group had a lower mean body mass index than did the dentate sample.

Thus, there are three areas of concern: first, that poor nutrition causes disease; second, that lack of teeth or painful teeth in young children may cause undernutrition and retarded growth; and, third, that an impaired dentition in elderly people results in undernutrition. However, before we can consider what advice to give, we need to consider what evidence there is on which to base the information.

It is useful to consider the evidence at three levels—each important.

- Does an impaired dentition affect food choice adversely?
- Does an impaired dentition affect nutrient intake and/or nutritional status?
- Does an impaired dentition affect health?

There is much evidence regarding food choice, some regarding nutrient intake or nutritional status, but virtually no evidence regarding health. This is a pity as health, after all, is the most relevant outcome. As we shall discover, food choice can be affected by an impaired dentition but does this result in malnutrition? Likewise, is a change in nutritional status clinically relevant?

# The impaired dentition, chewing ability, and food choice

## Case report

Jason, aged 10 years, is of short stature and is generally small for his age (Fig. 6.7). He has hypodontia and this lack of teeth—which, as he is in the mixed dentition stage, is not all that evident—coupled with a lack of occlusal contact, has made chewing difficult for him. Simple composite additions to the occlusal and incisal surfaces of the affected teeth will help.

There has been a sufficient number of studies published to conclude that the number of teeth lost is proportional to the difficulty that people have in eating foods and that this in turn affects food choice. Direct measurement of bite force and electromyographic methods have shown that people with dentures have much reduced bite force (only one fifth or one sixth that of dentate people) and that this is reduced further if dentures are uncomfortable. There is ample evidence that total loss of teeth and provision of complete dentures reduces the ability to break down foods for chewing or, alternatively, to get the same degree of food breakdown, more chewing strokes are needed. Chewing ability is closely correlated with the number of natural teeth present, and there appears to be a threshold of 20–21 teeth. Below this threshold, chewing ability declines, but above this figure loss of teeth has no apparent effect. These 20 teeth must occlude, so it is perhaps more accurate to say that there must be at least ten

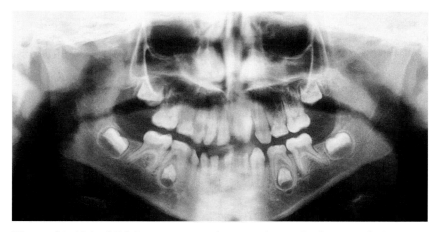

**Figure 6.7** This child (Jason; see text) has a syndrome the features of which include developmental delay and hypodontia. Lack of occlusion prevents him from chewing a variety of foods, which is his presenting complaint.

Table 6.1.
Problem foods for denture wearers

| Hard foods | Foods with seeds and small particles | Sticky foods |
|---|---|---|
| Meat, especially steak | Nuts | Chewing gum |
| Apples | Tomatoes | Fresh bread |
| Toast | Seeded jam | Sticky sweets, especially toffee |
| Bread crusts or rolls | Pears | Sticky cakes |
| Fresh fruit | Figs | Chocolate |
| Salads | Sugar | |
| Carrot | Grapes | |
| Celery | Coconut | |
| Corn on the cob | Rice | |
| | Caraway seeds | |
| | Peanut butter | |

Based on Ettinger (1973).

occluding pairs of teeth. In the most recent National Diet and Nutrition Survey (NDNS) conducted in 1995, of 955 people over 65 years, 12 per cent of free-living and 15 per cent of institutionalized people said eating was affected by their oral status. Of the two groups the latter were more likely to be edentulous.

If you ask a patient with full dentures what foods they find hard to eat, they will probably say apples and nuts. These anecdotal opinions are supported by the results of several studies which have enquired into food preferences in denture wearers. When the number of occasions foods were eaten by denture wearers was compared with dentate people, cheese and processed fruit were preferred by denture wearers, whereas salads, sandwiches, and raw vegetables were avoided by denture wearers. In the 1995 NDNS survey mentioned above, the impact of dental status on food choice was analysed in several ways—edentulousness, the number of natural teeth present, and the number of teeth occluding (number of occluding pairs of teeth). Regardless of the way dental status was classified, vegetables, fresh fruit, nuts, and meats were more difficult to eat for people with impaired dental status.

It is not only hard foods that are problem foods for denture wearers, but also foods with seeds and small particles (which get under dentures) and sticky foods (Table 6.1). Undoubtedly boiling vegetables and mincing meat increase their acceptability to denture wearers.

# The impaired dentition, diet, nutritional intake, and nutritional status

There have been far too few studies of nutrient intake and nutritional status of people in relation to their dental state and there is an especial shortage of well controlled studies. In the study of elderly people in Britain in 1967–8 already referred to, 13 per cent of the 700 subjects were judged to have 'insufficient mastication'. Not only did they have lower energy intake than those with 'efficient mastication' but they also ate 20 per cent less meat and 40 per cent less tomatoes, green vegetables, and raw non-citrus fruits. Three nutrients—energy, protein, and vitamin C—were of concern in those with 'insufficient mastication'.

A survey of nearly 400 elderly people in Sweden recorded lower protein and thiamine intakes in those with poor dentitions, after taking possible confounding factors (such as education, marital status, and income) into account. A survey in Finland found lower concentrations of serum pantothenic acid, ascorbic acid, and iron in those who were edentulous compared with dentate people. Fruit, vegetables, and 'fibre' intake was also reported to be lower in edentulous people in Canada.

The term 'non-starch polysaccharides' (NSP) is now preferred to 'dietary fibre'. Since fruit and vegetables are good sources of NSP, but are difficult for those with impaired dentition to chew, NSP is a risk nutrient. One of the first investigations into this was undertaken in the UK as recently as 1994. The edentulous group had a median NSP intake of 10.4 g/day, compared with a median of 15.1 g/day in the dentate group (Fig. 6.8), after matching for gender and social class. NSP intakes of 56 per cent of the edentulous group were below the current UK nutritional guidelines of 18 g/day. The dentate group obtained significantly more NSP from all the rich sources, such as wholemeal breads, cereals, vegetables, and fruit (Fig 6.9).

The 1995 National Diet and Nutrition Survey related nutrient intake to dental status. After statistical correction for the effects of age, gender, social class, and region, the mean daily intakes of NSP, protein, calcium, non-haem iron, niacin, vitamin C, and intrinsic and milk sugars were significantly lower in the

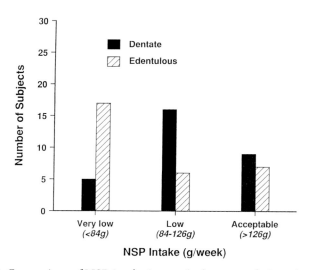

**Figure 6.8** Comparison of NSP intake in matched groups of edentulous and dentate adults. Reproduced with permission of *British Dental Journal*.

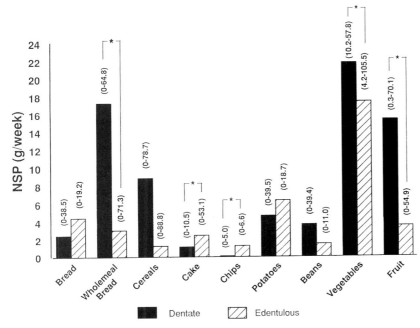

**Figure 6.9** Contribution of food sources to NSP intake in matched groups of edentulous and dentate adults. Reproduced with permission of *British Dental Journal*.

edentate adults. The same trends were also observed when dental status was expressed as 21 or more versus 20 or fewer teeth, or number of occluding pairs (OP) of teeth. Intake of NSP was particularly sensitive to the number of occluding pairs of teeth present—a mean of 13 g/day in those with no OP compared with 16 g/day for those with over five OP. Plasma iron concentration was lower in those with poor oral status, and edentate subjects had lower plasma levels of retinol, ascorbate, and $\alpha$-tocopherol compared with dentate subjects.

It seems quite clear that consumption of fruit and vegetables and intake of NSP are lower in edentulous persons. It is highly likely that this is a cause-and-effect relationship, but we cannot be sure since all the data presently available are from cross-sectional studies. A cause-and-effect relationship can only be established from longitudinal studies.

# The impaired dentition and health

There is little direct evidence that an impaired dentition causes ill health, but much indirect evidence that it is likely to do so. The exception is choking, which we will come to later.

The indirect evidence that an impaired dentition affects health is strong. Poor dental status affects food choice and dietary intake—fruit and vegetables, wholemeal bread, NSP are particularly at risk—and there is much evidence that low

**Box 6.1 Nutritional impact of poor dental status**

Risk nutrients
- Energy
- Protein
- Non-starch polysaccharides
- Iron
- Vitamins A, C, D

Risk foods
- 'Fibrous' foods
- Fresh fruit and vegetables
- Good quality meats

consumption of fruit, vegetables, and NSP increases the risk of a number of diseases—cancer of several organs, diverticular disease, and gallstones.

One fairly large Swedish study found that middle-aged edentulous men and women more often had two or more risk factors for cardiovascular disease compared with dentate persons, after the data were adjusted for the effects of gender and age. These factors included dietary habits—high fat and sugars intake and low vitamin intake—and smoking. In agreement with the finding of lower intake of NSP in dentally impaired persons, an American study found that such people took significantly more medication for gastrointestinal disturbances.

Choking on food is no joke. About 3000 people die in the USA per year from choking on food; it is the sixth most common cause of accidental death. In Canada, there are over 300 such deaths per year and, likewise in the UK, over 300 deaths per year are recorded for 'foreign bodies in the pharynx and larynx'—half of these in people over 65 years of age. There is likely to be considerable under-reporting of death by choking on food—for example, they are often recorded as 'café-coronary', since a survey of autopsies performed in all cases in which sudden death occurred during eating found a ratio of cases of food asphyxiation to occlusive coronary artery disease of 55:1.

So what has this to do with teeth? Well, quite a lot. There are at least nine publications which emphasize the role of poor dental health in food asphyxiation. A higher proportion of those choking to death on food were edentulous compared with the general population. The sizes of pieces of food responsible for death are frequently very large and usually show little evidence of mastication. Lack of intraoral sensation in those who wear full dentures has been mentioned by several authors as one reason for people attempting to swallow large unmasticated pieces of food.

From this rather fragmentary evidence, it seems that choking on food is a much more common cause of death than is usually thought, and lack of teeth seems likely to be a risk factor. Dentists and dietitians should warn edentulous elderly patients of the need to prepare food adequately for swallowing.

## The effect on nutrition of improving the dentition

Now that we know that loss of teeth is a risk factor for poor nutrition, we need to know whether improving the dentition results in improved food choice and nutrition. This has been looked at by a number of research teams in several countries. These studies are of two types—first, where poor-fitting complete dentures have been replaced by well-fitting complete dentures and, second, where fixed dental prostheses have replaced dentures. The results show that there was some improvement in chewing ability and food choice when the quality of complete dentures improved. In this respect, the fit of the lower denture was more important than the fit of the upper denture. However, it is surprising that, overall, providing fixed dental prostheses—with an osseointegrated oral implant bridge (OIB) or a tissue-integrated bridge (TIB)—in place of a removable denture did not improve chewing ability, food choice, or nutrient intake.

One important point when interpreting the above results is that dietary advice, on the whole, was not given at the same time as the dentures were improved. This is obviously of fundamental importance but has not been adequately tested. Improving the dentition alone is not enough—it is likely to be essential that good dietary advice is given at the same time. As Moynihan and colleagues have pointed out, not all foods rich in NSP are difficult to chew—dietary advice has to be personal, practical, and positive: these aspects will be discussed further in Chapters 8 and 10.

## Summary

- Teeth were essential for the survival of our ancestors, but modern food technology has meant that teeth are much less important for preparing food for swallowing and digestion than previously.

- Nutrition matters. Poor nutrition is an important cause of many diseases.

- An impaired dentition affects food choice—avoidance of fruit and vegetables in particular. There is also evidence that nutritional intake is adversely affected—lower consumption of fresh fruit and vegetables, NSP, and good quality meat.

- An impaired dentition is likely to affect health adversely, but evidence is indirect. However, choking on food is a significant cause of death, especially in the elderly.

- Improving an impaired dentition appears to lead to little improvement in food choice and nutrition. This may be because adequate dietary advice has not been given at the same time as an improvement in dental prostheses is made.

## Further reading

Brodeur, J. M., Laurin, D., Vallee, R., and Lachapelle, D. (1993). Nutrient intake and gastro-intestinal disorders related to masticatory performance in the edentulous elderly. *J. Prosthet. Dent.* **70**, 468–73.

Geissler, C. A. and Bates, J. E. (1984). The nutritional effects of tooth loss. *Am. J. Clin. Nutr.* **39**, 478–89.

Moynihan, P. J., Snow, S., Jepson, N. J. A., and Butler, T. J. (1994). Intake of non-starch polysaccharide (dietary fibre) in edentulous and dentate persons; an observational study. *Br. Dent. J.* **177**, 243–7.

Rugg-Gunn, A. J. (1993). *Nutrition and dental health*, Chapter 13. Oxford University Press, Oxford.

# 7

# Nutrition, diet, and oral health in children

# Nutrition, diet, and oral health in children

## Introduction

Despite the efforts of some sections of the food industry to muddy the waters, there has been very good agreement in the UK on nutritional messages for general health. It is important at any point in time that the best advice is put forward. This will mean that some advice may change when evidence is sufficiently strong to support the need for change. These changes have often been highlighted by the media, so that there is a danger that the public becomes confused. This confusion may be fuelled by misinformation from industries with vested interests. The reality is that the basic nutritional messages have changed very little—the purpose of the first part of this chapter is to summarize what this nutritional advice for general health is, before considering the more specific advice for oral health in children.

## Nutritional advice for general health

A number of authoritative, national reports have been published in the UK concerning children's nutrition and the more relevant are listed in Box 7.1. The most important policy document published in the UK in recent years has been the *Health of the nation*, published by the government in 1992. This spelt out

## Box 7.1 Chronological list of authoritative nutrition-related reports (most, but not all, are applicable to children)

| | |
|---|---|
| 1988 | *Present day practice in infant feeding: third report* (COMA) |
| 1989 | *Dietary sugars and human disease* (COMA) |
| 1991 | *Dietary reference values for food energy and nutrients for the United Kingdom* (COMA) |
| 1992 | *The nutrition of elderly people* (COMA) |
| | *Health of the nation* (government) |
| 1994 | *Eat well* (government) |
| | *Weaning and the weaning diet* (COMA) |
| | *Nutritional aspects of cardiovascular disease* (COMA) |
| 1996 | *Eat well II* (government) |
| | *The balance of good health* (HEA) |
| 1997 | *Healthy diets for infants and young children* (MAFF) |
| | *Our healthier nation* (government) |
| 1998 | Nutritional aspects of the development of cancer (COMA) |

quite clearly the major diseases and action required to reduce the impact of these diseases. Inevitably, dietary advice played a central part in this strategy as it is intimately involved in the major diseases—cardiovascular disease and cancer. In 1997, the new government in the UK published *Our healthier nation*, which continues with the same dietary messages. The very important point about both of these documents was that all departments in government—health, agriculture, education, employment—all agreed to the contents of the reports. The *Health of the nation* report had several spin-offs, of which the Nutrition Task Force is the most relevant to this discussion. The Nutrition Task Force produced two very useful policy documents: *Eat well* in 1994 and *Eat well II* in 1996.

The Nutrition Task Force publications refer to reports of the Committee on Medical Aspects of Food Policy (COMA). This is a standing committee in the Department of Health and has published a long list of excellent reports. The 1991 COMA report *Dietary reference values for food energy and nutrients for the UK* spelt out very clearly what nutrient intakes in the UK should be. It considered 40 nutrients and followed on from similar, but less comprehensive reports in 1969 and 1979. The 1991 recommendations are summarized in Table 7.1. Although the information is given for adults, it applies to children in broad terms. The report included separate chapters on sugars and starches. It proposed that the population's average intake of non-milk extrinsic sugars should not exceed about 60 g per day or 10 per cent of total dietary energy intake. Starches were grouped with intrinsic and milk sugars and these together should provide the main food energy requirements of the UK population.

Two years before the COMA dietary reference values report was published, COMA produced a report on *Dietary sugars and human disease*. The conclusions left no doubt that 'caries experience was positively related to the amount of non-milk extrinsic sugars in the diet and the frequency of their consumption'. One of the key recommendations is given in Box 7.2. The report also made a number of

## Box 7.2 From the COMA report Dietary sugars and human disease

In order to reduce the risk of dental caries, the Panel *recommends* that consumption of non-milk extrinsic sugars by the population should be decreased. These sugars should be replaced by fresh fruit, vegetables, and starchy foods.

## Table 7.1.

## Dietary reference values for fat and carbohydrate for adults as a percentage of daily total energy intake (percentage of food energy)

|  | Population average |
|---|---|
| Saturated fatty acids (maximum) | 10 (11) |
| Total fat (maximum) | 33 (35) |
| Non-milk extrinsic sugars (maximum) | 10 (11) |
| Intrinsic and milk sugars and starch (minimum) | 37 (39) |
| Total carbohydrate | 47 (50) |

The average percentage contribution to total energy does not total 100% because figures for protein and alcohol are excluded. Figures in parentheses apply when alcohol consumption is excluded from the calculations; this applies to children. Source: Department of Health (1991).

other relevant recommendations concerning more specific advice, which we will come to later.

The Department of Health COMA committee has produced at least three reports on infant feeding—the latest in 1988—key recommendations are given in Box 7.3. Following on from this, a report on 'Weaning and the weaning diet' was produced by COMA in 1994—important recommendations in this report are given in Box 7.4.

## Box 7.3 Some recommendations from the COMA report Present day practice in infant feeding: third report

- The Working Group reaffirms its earlier view that breastfeeding provides the best infant nutrition. We recommend that the Government Health Departments should encourage all healthy mothers to breastfeed their babies.
- In view of the lack of increase and the marked social class gradient in the prevalence of breastfeeding the Working Group recommends the search for new ways of encouraging breastfeeding especially in those sections of the community where it is shown to be low.
- We are concerned that breastfeeding has not yet gained complete social acceptance as the usual way of feeding babies. We urge social, community educational, commercial and other concerns to take a positive approach to this matter.
- We accept that, in the present climate of opinion about infant feeding, some mothers will choose to give infant formula feeds from birth and that the majority of infants will have received infant formula by the age of 4 weeks. We recommend that parents receive advice about infant formulas and about the preparation of feeds.
- Very few infants will require solid foods before the age of 3 months but the majority should be offered a mixed diet not later than the age of 6 months. We recommend accordingly.
- We recommend that breastfeeding or feeding with infant formula can, with advantage, be continued to at least the end of the first year as part of a mixed diet.
- We recommend that fully skimmed cow's milk, because of its low energy density and vitamin A content, is not suitable in the diet of the under 5 year old. Semi-skimmed milk may, in certain circumstances, be included in the diet of the child over 2 years.
- We recommend that infants should receive vitamin supplements, as advised.
- Vitamin supplementation. The Working Party recommends that the Government should continue to make supplementary vitamins for infants and young children available. The daily dose should be 5 drops which will contain approximately

  vitamin A    200 µg
  vitamin C    20 mg
  vitamin D    7 µg
- We recommend that vitamin supplementation should be given to infants and young children aged from 6 months up to at least 2 years and preferably 5 years.

## Box 7.4 Some recommendations from the COMA report Weaning and the weaning diet

- The majority of infants should not be given solid foods before the age of 4 months, and a mixed diet should be offered by the age of 6 months.
- Infants should be supervised during mealtimes. Semi-solid food should be given from a spoon and not mixed with milk or other drink in a bottle. From 6 months of age, infants should be introduced to drinking from a cup and from age 1 year feeding from a bottle should be discouraged.
- For groups of children the average intake of non-milk extrinsic sugars should be limited to about 10 per cent of total dietary energy intake.
- Adequate vitamin status should be encouraged for mother and baby through a varied diet and moderate exposure to summer sunlight.
- Between the ages of 1 and 5 years, vitamin A and D supplements should be given unless adequate vitamin status can be assured from a diverse diet containing vitamins A- and D-rich foods and from moderate exposure to sunlight.
- Milk (also including breast milk, infant formula, follow-on formula) or water should constitute the majority of the total drinks given. Other drinks should usually be confined to mealtimes and because of the risk to dental health, they should not be given in a feeding bottle or at bedtime.
- Non-wheat cereals, fruit, vegetables, and potatoes are suitable first weaning foods. Salt should not be added and additional sugars should be limited to that needed for palatability of sour fruits. Between 6 and 9 months of age the amount and variety of foods including meat, fish, eggs, all cereals, and pulses should be increased and the number of 'milk' feeds reduced. Food consistency should progress from puréed through minced/mashed to finely chopped. By the age of 1 year the diet should be mixed and varied.
- In the later states of weaning, three meals per day are suggested with two or three snacks in addition.
- Infants and young children who are failing to thrive should be identified as early as possible, and a nutritional cause should be investigated.
- Weaning foods should usually be free of, or low in, non-milk extrinsic sugars including sugars derived from fruit juices and fruit concentrates. The range of commercial foods meeting these criteria should be increased. Foods and drinks which predispose to caries should be limited to main mealtimes. The sugars content of all weaning foods and drinks should be shown on food labels.
- Water supplies should be fluoridated to the optimum of one part per million. For infants and young children in areas that are not fluoridated, fluoride supplements may be advised where there is a particular risk of caries.
- Professional staff who advise parents about weaning should be trained and should have access to dietetic expertise.

Three more COMA reports, which concern adults more than children, are relevant: *Nutrition of elderly people*, published in 1992; *Nutritional aspects of cardiovascular disease*, published in 1994; and *Nutritional aspects of the development of cancer*, published in 1998. All made important recommendations for improving diet for general health and will be discussed further in Chapter 8.

The messages from these several reports are quite clear. We need to increase our consumption of staple starchy foods, fresh fruit and vegetables and reduce our consumption of fat and sugars. Special recommendations apply to infants and young children and to elderly people.

Although nutritional advice is given in terms of nutrients (as it is these which influence health and disease), what people actually eat are foods, so practical advice has to be given in terms of foods. This translation of nutrient requirements into food recommendations has been made very successfully by the Health Education Authority (HEA) in their programme 'The balance of good health'. This is reproduced in Fig. 7.1. This pictorial representation of what constitutes a balanced diet has been very carefully thought out. It is not the only model of its kind, but it has been widely accepted as most useful in helping health professionals to give dietary advice to the general public. The knife and fork are important, indicating that meals, as opposed to on-the-hoof snacks, are highly desirable.

The five segments represent five food groups and vary in size according to the contribution which these groups should make to achieving a balanced diet. The proportion is as follows:

- bread, other cereals, and potatoes: 33 per cent;
- fruit and vegetables: 33 per cent;
- milk and dairy foods: 15 per cent;
- meat, fish, and alternatives: 12 per cent; and
- foods containing fat and/or foods containing sugar: 8 per cent.

Box 7.5 gives the key characteristics of foods within each of the five groups.

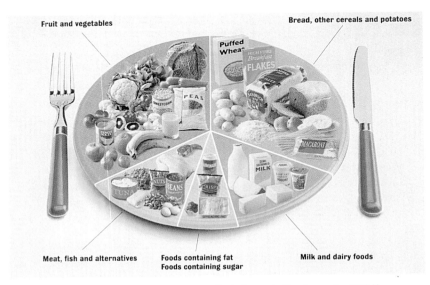

**Figure 7.1** A pictorial representation of a balanced diet from the HEA's programme 'The balance of good health'.

## Box 7.5 'The balance of good health'

The key characteristics of foods within each of the five groups are described below.

### Bread, other cereals, and potatoes
- major sources of starchy carbohydrate and non-starch polysaccharide (NSP)
- predominantly low in fat and can be consumed without the addition of fat
- commonly consumed, readily available, affordable and with transcultural application
- key nutrients: carbohydrate, NSP, vitamin B complex, calcium, and iron

### Fruit and vegetables
- major source of vitamins, minerals, and NSP
- commonly consumed, readily available, affordable and with transcultural application
- key nutrients: range of vitamins, minerals, NSP, and carbohydrate

### Milk and dairy foods
- frequently contribute to calcium intake
- lower fat alternatives available and encouraged
- commonly consumed, readily available, affordable and with transcultural application
- key nutrients: major source of calcium, protein, vitamin $B_{12}$, vitamins A, D, and E

### Meat, fish, and alternatives
- frequently contribute to iron intake
- major source of protein
- can be low in fat (particularly saturated fat) or reduced fat alternatives available
- commonly consumed, readily available, affordable and with transcultural application
- key nutrients: major source of protein, iron, B vitamins, zinc, magnesium, and (from pulses only) NSP

### Foods containing fat; foods containing sugar
- principal source of energy as fat or sugar or combination of fat and sugar
- key nutrients:
    from fat—essential, fat-soluble vitamins, but chiefly a source of energy
    from sugar—chiefly a source of energy

Health Education Authority (1996).

## Box 7.6 Other briefing papers from the HEA

*Diet and cancer*
*Diet and health in school age children*
*Dietary fats*
*Nutritional aspects of cardiovascular disease*
*Nutrition in minority ethnic groups*
*Obesity and overweight*
*Scientific basis of nutrition education*
*Starch and dietary fibre*
*Sugars in the diet*

The Health Education Authority has produced a number of excellent publications informing health professionals what nutritional messages should be. All this advice is clearly based on COMA recommendations. The HEA has produced a very readable series of 'briefing papers' which are strongly recommended and listed in Box 7.6.

A useful guide for nutrition educators is *Eight guidelines for a healthy diet* published in 1997. It gives practical advice on eating and drinking sensibly and, most importantly, enjoying food. This last point is tremendously important. Dietary advice shouldn't be seen as negative; eating should be a normal and pleasurable experience. Helping people to want to make sensible dietary choices is vital and the dental team has an important role to make this so.

The Ministry of Agriculture, Fisheries and Foods (MAFF) has also produced helpful publications to advise health professionals—for example *Healthy diets for infants and young children*. The advice is practical, covering aspects such as fussy eaters, breakfasts, and food allergies, as well as two pages of useful addresses for further advice (e.g. the La Leche League and the Vegetarian Society).

Foods and drinks provided in schools have been a continuing area of concern for many years. Many people believe that quality has declined along with popularity—by the early 1990s less than half of school children ate school meals. To try to help schools improve the quality of foods they offer, the Caroline Walker Trust published *Nutritional guidelines for school meals* in 1992.

Thus, it can be seen that there is no shortage of advice for healthy eating for general health in the UK. What is very important is that it is consistent. This has very largely been achieved, as there is agreement between government departments, professions, and between specialities within professions—for example, the medical, dental, and dietetic professions. Now we consider advice for oral health for each age group in turn, bearing in mind points of advice for general health discussed in the first part of this chapter. The evidence for the following advice was discussed in Chapters 2 to 5.

# Advice for oral health of children and young people

## Pregnancy and the neonatal period

### Malnutrition and vitamin D

In countries with generally adequate levels of nutrition, nutrition during pregnancy is thought to have little influence on the future dental health of the unborn child. For example, the Health Education Authority in its latest policy document states:

> Some teeth are more resistant to attack than others, but there is nothing from the nutritional point of view, fluoride apart, that can be done about this. Contrary to popular belief neither malnutrition in mother during pregnancy, nor in the child after birth, is likely to have any appreciable effect on the susceptibility of teeth to decay. Calcium cannot be removed from the mother's teeth by the foetus during pregnancy or due to lactation. Fluoride is the only factor that has been shown, beyond doubt, to decrease susceptibility to decay. The effect of fluoride is due partly to its incorporation into the developing tooth before its eruption into the mouth and partly to its direct contact with the tooth after eruption. The latter is now thought to be the more important.

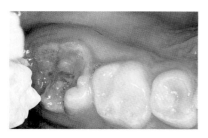

**Figure 7.2** Severe enamel hypoplasia of a first permanent molar tooth in a child born prematurely and who had a 'stormy' neonatal period.

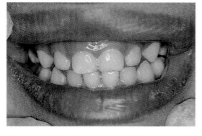

**Figure 7.3** Fluorosis of the enamel of the incisal half of teeth 52 and 51. Reproduced with permission of Dr M Malik.

Certainly the above document is right to emphasize that the post-eruptive effect of sugars in the diet is of paramount importance, but there are sufficient data, reviewed in Chapters 2 and 3, to indicate that even in some industrialized countries, nutrition while the teeth are forming is of some relevance.

In areas with high prevalence of malnutrition, enamel formed before birth is adversely affected, with a higher occurrence of hypoplasia, although the severity of hypoplasia is greater in enamel formed neonatally and postnatally (Fig. 7.2). Dental caries experience is positively related to the presence of enamel hypoplasia and malnutrition, and it is reasonable to assume that some, although probably a small proportion, of these adverse events lead to an increased susceptibility to dental caries.

It should be remembered from Chapter 2 that the study of Cockburn and others in Edinburgh, UK, showed clear relationships between provision of vitamin D supplements during pregnancy and lower prevalence of hypocalcaemia in infants and lower prevalence of hypoplastic primary teeth when the children were 2–3 years of age. A study in London reported a strong relationship between low birthweight and occurrence of hypoplasia in primary teeth. Although causes of low birthweight were not given, poor nutrition is likely to have been a factor. Thus, there is some evidence that nutritional deficiencies, and vitamin D in particular in pregnancy, can cause enamel hypoplasia and thus predispose to caries in the primary dentition. Vitamin D supplementation remains desirable for all pregnant and lactating women. On present evidence this seems likely to benefit the primary dentition of at least some children.

### Fluoride

A number of studies have investigated the effect of fluoride given prenatally on the subsequent caries experience of the child. These studies are difficult to interpret with much authority. However, it is reasonable to conclude that there is likely to be a small benefit to the child but that the size of this benefit is too small to warrant recommending fluoride supplements during pregnancy.

Excessive ingestion of fluoride during pregnancy can result in fluorosis of enamel formed prenatally in the child's primary dentition (Fig. 7.3). The placenta acts as quite an effective barrier to fluoride so that ingestion has to be very high to produce enamel fluorosis: as an example, cases have been recorded in areas of Sweden receiving drinking water containing 5–10 mg F/l of water. Other nutritional deficiencies or excesses have not been associated with intraoral congenital abnormalities, with the exception perhaps of a possible relationship between folic acid deficiency and clefts of lip and palate.

## Dental health of the mother

Of some concern is the oral health of the mother during pregnancy. Pregnancy gingivitis is a well recognized event and is characterized by hyperaemia and swollen gingivae which bleed during brushing or even eating. Removal of dental calculus and good plaque control by tooth brushing will do much to reduce its occurrence and severity. Remission occurs post-partum. A number of clinical trials, conducted mainly in New Zealand, have reported reductions in pregnancy gingivitis in women using folate mouth-rinses. This treatment, which may be termed local nutrition, is not used widely.

Dietary habits can change significantly during pregnancy, but the time period is probably too short to have a great impact on dental caries. Likewise, vomiting as a cause of erosion during pregnancy has not been seen as a great threat to dental health. Advice to limit the frequency of consumption of sugar-containing snacks is sensible for the health of the mother.

## Infancy and weaning

Diet and nutrition are relevant to dental health during the first year of life in two ways. First, the pre-eruptive effect—the deciduous dentition continues to develop within the jaws and calcification of the permanent dentition begins. Malnutrition can cause the formation of hypoplastic enamel and increase susceptibility to dental caries. Good general nutrition is therefore of some significance to both dentitions. These deficiencies are thought by most people to be only relevant to developing nations, but good data showing that they are irrelevant in developed countries are lacking. Vitamin supplementation (usually a combination of vitamins A, C, and D) is recommended for infants and young children in the UK and is likely to benefit the future oral and dental health of some children (Box 7.3).

Second, the first teeth erupt at about 6 months (with considerable variation) and the frequency and duration of exposure of these newly erupted teeth to sugars **in foods consumed** is very important in determining whether or not they develop caries; this is much more important than any pre-eruptive **nutritional** effect.

Milk is of very low cariogenicity if extra sugar is not added. The dental profession rightly encourages breastfeeding, as breastfed babies tend to have lower dental caries experience than bottle-fed babies, probably because of the lack of opportunity to add sugar to feeds and the lower use of reservoir feeders and comforters containing sugary fruit-flavoured drinks. The development of dental caries is only associated with breastfeeding when it is prolonged (over 1 year) and on demand and even then, dental caries is uncommon.

The addition of sucrose to milk in bottles to prevent constipation is still widespread, especially among new immigrant groups. Two thirds of Asian mothers living in Leeds, UK, added sugars to the milk-based feeds of their infants. These parents strongly believed that the addition of sugar was good for their child. Thus, health education has a considerable way to go to ensure that extra sugar is not added to bottle feeds.

The strong relationship between sugar-containing fruit-flavoured drinks used as a comforter in a bottle or reservoir feeder and the development of dental caries (Figs 7.4 and 7.5) was emphasized in Chapter 3. In a recent survey, it was reported that 18 per cent of pre-school children used a dinky or reservoir feeder, from which nearly 40 per cent consumed sweetened juice. Authoritative committees have repeatedly urged that these drinks should not be used as a comforter and that thirsty children will drink water. Giving sugary drinks (or foods) just before the infant or child goes to sleep is likely to be especially damaging because the favourable flow of saliva virtually ceases during sleep. In addition,

Box 7.8

Winter, commenting on the role of the sweetened feeding bottle as a cause of dental caries in young children, said: 'The fashion throughout this century of mothers substituting the nursing bottle for the maternal breast has played a significant part in this respect'.

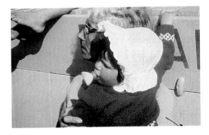

**Figure 7.4** A child using a reservoir feeder containing sweetened fruit juice.

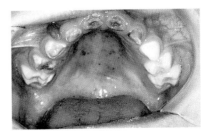

**Figure 7.5** The intraoral view of the child from Fig. 7.4 showing the extensive carious destruction as a result of the feeder habit.

Box 7.9

Mothers of first babies, aged less than 1 year, reported that 43 per cent of their babies were breastfed, 21 per cent were given milk in a bottle with no added sugar, while 36 per cent were given milk in a bottle with sugar added. Of those who added sugar to milk, 62 per cent said that this had been advised by the hospital staff or the health visitor.

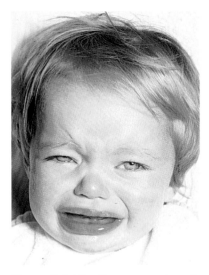

**Figure 7.6** The distress experienced by a child who is teething.

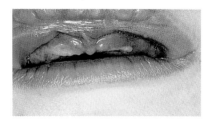

**Figure 7.7** An intraoral view of the child in Fig. 7.6 showing the erupting maxillary primary incisors—the cause of the distress.

reliance on sweetened drinks by toddlers often dulls the appetite and inadequate nutrition is the consequence—now termed 'squash-bottle syndrome'!

Provision of fluoride will help the forming teeth as well as teeth which have just erupted into the mouth. If the fluoride concentration in the drinking water is low, fluoride supplements can be recommended, but most authorities suggest that these should not begin before the age of 6 months. Teeth should be brushed with a toothpaste suitable for young children (Box 7.10).

Teething can be troublesome in infancy (Figs 7.6 and 7.7): over 50 per cent of pre-school children are reported to have trouble teething. Diet and nutrition have little influence on teething, but chewing on hard foods can bring relief. (Fig. 7.8)

The importance of good feeding practices in the first year of life has been emphasized by many people who have demonstrated that dietary patterns are established during this first year, and that patterns of behaviour learnt at this time are very resistant to change subsequently. As many of our attitudes and habits concerning food and health are acquired during this period of primary socialization, it is essential that health education should start with pregnant and nursing mothers.

## Box 7.10 Appropriate fluoride prescribing for children

| Age | mg F per day |
|---|---|
| 6 months up to 3 years | 0.25 |
| 3 up to 6 years | 0.50 |
| 6 years and over | 1.00 |

Notes

1. In areas with water supplies containing fluoride at or above 0.3 ppm F dentists should consider a lower dosage. This would mean that where the water fluoride concentration was between 0.3 and 0.7 mg F/l, no supplements are given to children less than 3 years; between 3 and 6 years, 0.25 mg F/day can be given; and over 6 years, 0.5 mg F/day. No supplements are recommended where water supplies contain more than 0.7 mg F/l.

2. To reduce the risk of opacities, children under the age of 6 years and considered to be at low risk of developing dental caries should use a toothpaste containing no more than 600 ppm of fluoride. Those with a higher risk of developing caries should use a standard (1000 ppm) paste. Children over the age of 6 should be encouraged to use a standard (1000 ppm) or higher (1450 ppm) fluoride level paste. Toothpastes accredited by the British Dental Association should be recommended.

3. Children under 6 years old should use an amount of toothpaste no greater than a small pea. Formal recommendations should emphasize *small*, rather than rely simply on *pea-sized* amount, which may be too much. To reduce the risk of opacities, parents must supervise the amount of toothpaste used during brushing up to the age of 6 years. Help with or close supervision of brushing up to at least 7 or 8 years is recommended to ensure effective plaque removal.

British Society of Paediatric Dentistry (1996).

## Box 7.11  Teething

Teething is most usually associated with the imminent eruption of primary lower incisors, commonly between about 4 and 8 months. The infant is fretful and the cheeks may be red. Intraorally the gums may be red (Fig. 7.7). Relief can be obtained by biting on something hard, such as a clean teething ring. Such objects should be too large to enter the mouth to avoid the chance of choking or swallowing. Hard foods can be given; rusks may be better than carrots or apple slices since rusks will dissolve, lessening the risk of choking. Analgesics (paracetamol) can be prescribed and parents reassured.

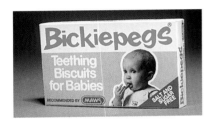

**Figure 7.8** Hard, sugar-free teething rusks can bring relief to the teething child.

## Box 7.12  Key points—infancy

- Pre-eruptive effect of nutrition on permanent teeth
- Adding sugar to bottles
- Sugary fruit-flavoured drinks
- Fluoride
- Teething

If solid foods are taken at usual mealtimes only, then the risk of dental caries is small. The problem arises when sugary foods are given frequently and chief among the culprits are confectionery and biscuits. The most popular reason for mothers giving their young child confectionery is 'reward for good behaviour', while the second most important reason is to 'pacify the child'. The poster produced by the Health Education Authority (Fig. 7.9) conveys this message with style.

## The pre-school child

Feeding practices in infancy have been a major influence on dental caries experience in pre-school children, as emphasized in the previous section. Nevertheless, dental caries continues to occur at the ages of 2, 3, and 4 years. About half of 5 year olds have caries experience in the UK and this figure has remained stable for about 10 years. In the emerging nations of the Middle East and Far East, caries experience in pre-school children is very high with over 80 per cent of 5 year olds affected. In a survey of 5 year olds in Abu Dhabi in 1996, the mean dmft was 8.3—over one third of primary teeth affected by caries.

There are little data on the sugar intake of pre-school children. In one survey in the UK, sugar provided 22 per cent of energy intake. Between-meal snacking is prevalent and most pre-school children have snacks at mid-morning and mid-afternoon: sweet biscuits are the most important food, and milk and fruit squash the most popular drinks. Over half of toddlers in the UK have a drink in bed at

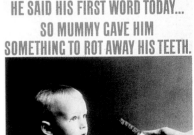

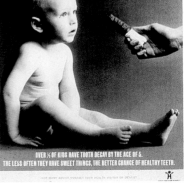

**Figure 7.9** The HEA's poster depicting the use of confectionery as a 'reward'. Reproduced with permission of the Health Education Authority.

Box 7.13 **Key points—young child**

- High sugar snacks
- Fluoride
- Attendances at dentist
- Liquid oral medicines

night, usually milk or sweetened juice. Pre-school children from manual worker backgrounds were more likely to be given sugar confectionery and carbonated drinks daily. Likewise, double the proportion of households from manual backgrounds spent more than £5 on confectionery per week, compared with families from non-manual backgrounds—11 per cent and 5 per cent respectively.

Fluoride has an important role in prevention of caries in the pre-school child. An adequate level of fluoride in drinking water has a marked beneficial effect on caries experience in the primary dentition. This effect is largely topical—a local action on teeth which have erupted into the mouth—although some systemic (pre-eruptive) effect on the primary dentition can be identified. Many permanent teeth are forming in the pre-school years and fluoride can provide a useful pre-eruptive effect in these teeth. In the absence of adequate levels of fluoride in the water, dietary supplements of fluoride can be given—the dosage depending on the fluoride content of drinking water and on the age of the child (Box 7.10). Drops are usually used up to the age of 2 years (often combined with vitamin supplements in the USA) and these can be given either in a spoon or in food and water, as long as all the food or water is ingested. Over the age of 2 years, the daily fluoride tablet can be sucked to produce a topical effect in the mouth before swallowing: the tablet should be moved around the mouth to ensure good distribution of fluoride. The teeth of pre-school children should be brushed with a suitable fluoride-containing toothpaste (Box 7.10).

It is important to realize that both tooth-brushing with a fluoride-containing toothpaste and sugar control are important in caries prevention in the pre-school child. Although in reality, good tooth-brushing habits and good dietary habits go hand in hand, many studies have shown that both independently contribute to dental health, and both tooth-brushing and diet should be emphasized if oral health of children is to be optimal.

The age at which a child first attends a dentist for examination varies, but most paediatric dentists believe that it should be as early as possible to use the opportunity for practical dietary advice around the time of weaning and thereafter. Such early attendance is encouraged by the method by which dentists are paid in the general dental service where babies can be registered for care. There is no reason why a parent and child should not attend for advice before this age and, indeed, this is actively encouraged in the USA and Scandinavia.

The problem of dietary erosion of teeth would seem to be a prevalent problem in young children and should be looked for specifically during examination of the pre-school child. The most recent National Diet and Nutrition Survey of pre-school children reported that half the children in this age group had some evidence of erosion. This may well indicate a potential risk for the permanent dentition.

Many children take medicines and, for young children, these are often given in a liquid form. The damaging effect of the frequent use of sugar-containing liquid oral medicines is well known and the advantages of non-sugar sweeteners in these medicines is clear. In the UK, it is regrettable that still 60 per cent of liquid oral medicines are sugar-based. Those who care for children and advise parents should ensure that sugar-free preparations are selected (Fig. 7.10).

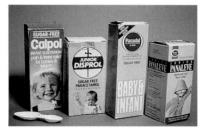

**Figure 7.10** A selection of sugar-free paracetamol preparations suitable for children.

# The school child and adolescent

Between the ages of 6 and 12 years is the period of the 'mixed dentition'—when primary teeth are shed and replaced by their permanent successors. The local intraoral effect of dietary sugars is of greatest importance but the role of nutrition on forming teeth cannot be dismissed completely.

Dietary fluoride continues to be important throughout the years of childhood and adolescence. Whether in drinking water, salt, milk, or as dietary supplements, fluoride is incorporated into permanent teeth which are still forming and, more importantly, provides a topical caries-preventive effect on newly erupted permanent teeth at a time when they are (1) most susceptible to dental decay, and (2) still undergoing post-eruptive maturation. While the amount of fluoride ingested should be limited (so that fluoride dietary supplements are not given in areas with an optimum level of fluoride in the drinking water, for example), any number of topical fluoride agents (e.g. toothpaste, mouth-rinses, gels, varnishes) can be used, if the risk of dental caries warrants it.

There are little data on the diets of school children aged 5–10 years, partly due to the difficulties of collection at this age, but there is much more information on the diets of adolescents. Adolescence is the time of rapid growth, independent food choices, and food fads. As with adults, children and adolescents in the UK consume diets which contain too much fat (providing about 40 per cent of dietary energy instead of about 35 per cent) and too little starch, non-starch polysaccharides (fruit and vegetables), iron, and calcium. Fairly comprehensive data are available for sugars intake in adolescent children. All sugars provide about 21 per cent of energy intake. Of this, 30 per cent comes from intrinsic and milk sugars (i.e. from fruit and vegetables, providing about 20 per cent, and milk, about 10 per cent) of this total sugars intake. The remaining 70 per cent of sugars intake comes from non-milk extrinsic sugars. Intrinsic and milk sugars are not a threat to teeth and are part of desirable food groups (fruit, vegetables, and milk products): consumption of these foods should be encouraged. The 1991 COMA report on dietary reference values grouped intrinsic and milk sugars with starch, and recommended that this group should provide most of dietary energy. On the other hand, non-milk extrinsic sugars have repeatedly been shown to be the main dietary cause of caries and, on the whole, are consumed in less desirable foods—such as confectionery: the consumption of these foods should be limited to mealtimes and occasional treats (Fig. 7.1, Box 7.5).

A third of non-milk extrinsic sugars comes from confectionery and over 80 per cent of non-milk extrinsic sugars from just four sources—confectionery, table sugar, soft drinks, and biscuits and cakes. None of these are nutritionally desirable foods but they are heavily advertised, easy to eat anywhere, anytime, and popular. Not only is confectionery the main source of sugars and the second source of dietary fats in children, but it is made and advertised for frequent eating and is often sticky, delaying oral clearance. Not surprisingly, the dental profession has singled out confectionery for special criticism in dental health education.

International comparisons can be interesting. American children consume more sugars than English children, but the sources of sugars are quite different

(Table 7.2). While 36 per cent of sugars come from confectionery and table sugar and 18 per cent from milk and fruit in English children, the percentages are reversed in American children with 18 per cent coming from confectionery and table sugar and 31 per cent from milk and fruit. In simple terms, English children eat twice as much confectionery but only half as much fruit and much less milk than American children.

A multitude of factors govern our choice of food, such as availability, costs, traditions, culture, taste, and emotions. Apart from a general reduction in intake, options to reduce intake include eating confectionery at one time in the week only—the 'Saturday sweets' idea has made considerable progress in Scandinavia—and substitution of sugars by non-sugar sweeteners. Dietary habits are often difficult to change and methods of doing so will be considered further in Chapter 10.

The last nutritional aspect of dental health of children to consider is erosion. Because of the rise in consumption of soft drinks—just look at easy access to vending machines in schools—it is likely to be a growing problem. Apart from acid drinks, frequent regurgitation occurs in children due to a variety of causes, including anorexia nervosa. Prevention is important, as treatment is often difficult and expensive. Establishing the cause, if erosion is suspected, can be difficult, but is important if prevention and, if necessary, treatment, are to be successful. Reducing the frequency of drinking acidic drinks and reducing the time for which they contact the teeth, perhaps by using a straw, are important goals. In difficult cases, but with a cooperative patient, mouth-guards may be desirable—especially for nocturnal vomiters. Fluoride is thought to reduce erosion.

An important motivating factor is appearance, which many adolescents are obsessive about: this will be discussed further in connection with dietary advice in Chapter 10.

Table 7.2.

Comparison of the mean daily intake of dietary sugars by 11–12-year-old American and English children

| Source | USA 143 g (24% energy) % | | England 118 g (21% energy) % | |
|---|---|---|---|---|
| Milk | 20 | } 31 | 13 | } 18 |
| Fruit (excluding juice) | 11 | | 5 | |
| Confectionery | 8 | } 18 | 19 | } 36 |
| Table sugar | 10 | | 17 | |
| Soft drinks (including juice[a]) | 23 | | 14 | |

[a] Not possible to separate data into fresh fruit juices and other soft drinks.

## The sick child

Two aspects of dietary advice for oral health are of concern for the sick child. First, the diseases themselves may require special diets which may or may not be favourable to dental health and, second, dental disease can be a considerable threat to patients with some diseases. Thus, prevention of dental disease, through dietary means, is especially important for these patients. If total sugar intake is included within this discussion, then sugared medicines should be considered, since they are likely to be used daily, long term, in some of these patients. The potential for some medicines to be erosive should also be considered (Table 7.3).

Diseases which require special diets can be considered under two broad headings—those in which diet is an essential part of the treatment of their chronic disorder (for example, coeliac disease, phenylketonuria, cystic fibrosis) and those in which medical and dental implications may occur if diet is not considered as part of overall care (for example, diabetes). Patients suffering from inborn errors of metabolism (for example, phenylketonuria, maple syrup urine disease) or fat metabolism (for example, abetalipoproteinaemia) are likely to require high carbohydrate diets. This also applies to other inborn errors of metabolism (such as cystic fibrosis) while a number of inborn errors of carbohydrate metabolism require a change of carbohydrate (such as lactose or fructose intolerance).

It is vital that those who care for these patients are aware of these special dietary needs and consult with the patient's physician or dietitian before offering dietary advice. High carbohydrate diets have to be attractive to the patient—and this may well mean high sugar content—and may have to be taken frequently. In such cases, a dentist needs to use all other available means—fluorides, plaque control, and fissure sealing—to prevent dental caries. Remember that patients with phenylketonuria should not consume the non-sugar sweetener aspartame, as

Box 7.15

'Casual though well-meaning statements to omit sugar from a child's diet can lead—in a case where it is medically required, such as certain inborn errors of metabolism—to growth failure, weight loss, biochemical instability, and can even be life-threatening. After all, it is no good having a good dentition in the grave.' A leading paediatric dietitian.

Table 7.3.

## The endogenous pH and titratable acidity of some oral liquid medicines and effervescent tablets

| Sample | pH | Titratable acidity[a] |
|---|---|---|
| Potassium chloride 7.5% syrup | 6.0 | 0.02 |
| Hydralazine suspension 5 mg/5 ml | 2.6 | 1.54 |
| Propranolol suspension 5 mg/5 ml | 2.8 | 0.05 |
| Lactulose solution 3.35 mg/5 ml | 4.6 | 0.01 |
| Senokot syrup 7.5 mg/5 ml | 5.4 | 0.03 |
| Amoxycillin suspension 7.5 mg/5 ml | 6.3 | 0.05 |
| Cephalexin suspension 125 mg/5 ml | 5.2 | 0.85 |
| Phosphate-Sandoz tablet | 4.6 | 10.66 |
| Sando-K tablet | 3.5 | 8.39 |
| Captopril suspension 5 mg/5 ml | 3.7 | 0.03 |

[a] ml of 0.1 N NaOH.

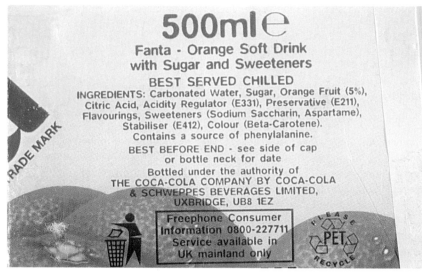

Figure 7.11 A label from a can of carbonated orange drink showing the warning 'Contains a source of phenylalanine'.

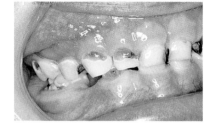

Figure 7.12 An intraoral view of the mouth of a child with asthma who has received a constant supply of sweetened medicines as well as sugary fruit drinks.

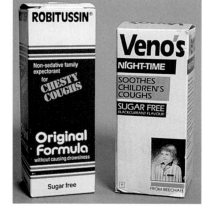

Figure 7.13 Sugar-free liquid oral medicines.

it contains the amino acid phenylalanine (Fig. 7.11) and that patients with hereditary fructose intolerance should not be prescribed sucrose- or fructose-containing medicines. Some scope for change of the diet may be possible, for example the timing of foods or medicines, and discussion between dentist and physician or dietitian, can help the patient.

The second group of patients are those whose life may be at risk from poor oral health. This group includes patients in whom sepsis is hazardous (e.g. congenital or acquired heart defects, renal disorders, patients with prostheses, immune deficiency diseases), general anaesthesia is hazardous (cardiac diseases, asthma) (Fig. 7.12), and patients with disorders of haemostasis (haemophiliacs, etc.). These patients should be selected for special preventive care which will include dietary advice for the prevention of oral and dental diseases.

The problem of sugared medicines has been discussed earlier in this chapter. About 1 in 800 children take sugared medicines daily, long term. Less than half the liquid oral medicines used long term by children in the UK are sugar-free and those who prescribe for these patients, pharmacists who sell medicines, and parents who buy medicines should be aware of the non-cariogenic alternatives (Fig. 7.13).

# Some factors which influence the diets of children

## Parents and grandparents

Mothers usually have the greatest influence on the child's diet. Early in life the mother is likely to be the sole provider and habits formed early tend to last. Good and bad dietary habits tend to be passed from parent to child. Mothers who add sugar to their coffee are much more likely to add sugar to their baby's milk. In a survey in Edinburgh, 75 per cent of mothers usually gave their child sweets after nursery school—19 per cent gave them as a reward, 24 per cent to keep the child quiet, and 57 per cent because the child demanded sweets. Nutrition was not a reason.

Sweets are frequently given as a reward and seen as a token of affection. Grandparents are often considered to be a significant source of confectionery for young children, although data supporting this are difficult to find. Likewise, child-minders are occasionally thought to buy peace with confectionery but, again, this is largely anecdotal opinion. It should be borne in mind that a significant number of pre-school children will be looked after by someone other than a parent (Table 7.4) and that these carers should be aware of the dietary advice you are giving.

It is also important to recognize that a great many parents take good care of their child's diet and are rightly sensitive to criticism. Praise should be given wherever possible.

## Hospitals and health visitors

In the past, hospital staff and health visitors frequently recommended the addition of sugar to bottle-feeds for infants as a cure for constipation or just for 'comfort' (Box 7.9). Now this practise is discouraged, it is hoped that it will become less prevalent.

## Social class

Patterns of sugar eating in young children are strongly related to social class. Breastfeeding is less common in social classes IV and V (unskilled workers) while the addition of sugar to bottles and the use of reservoir feeders are more common

## Table 7.4.
## Pattern of child care for pre-school children

|  | Age of child (years) | | | |
|---|---|---|---|---|
|  | $1\frac{1}{2}-2\frac{1}{2}$ | $2\frac{1}{2}-3\frac{1}{2}$ | $3\frac{1}{2}-4\frac{1}{2}$ | All ages |
|  | % | % | % | % |
| Mother not working | 62 | 57 | 56 | 58 |
| Mother working and child looked after by |  |  |  |  |
| Mother | 5 | 5 | 3 | 4 |
| Father | 12 | 16 | 13 | 14 |
| Other relative | 11 | 12 | 13 | 12 |
| Paid childminder | 6 | 5 | 4 | 5 |
| Other[a] | 3 | 5 | 10 | 6 |

[a] Includes day nursery, creche, play group, and nursery school.
National Diet and Nutrition Survey (1995).

in social classes IV and V than in social classes I and II (professional and managerial workers).

In a study of the sweet-eating habits of nursery school children in Edinburgh, mothers in deprived areas of the city were more likely to give their 3–4 year old children sweets after school, using sweets as comforters, spend more money on sweets, and allow sweet consumption throughout the day than mothers in non-deprived areas. Children in deprived areas had more than three times more dental decay than children in the non-deprived areas, in line with national trends. Social class trends in sugar consumption are much less marked in adolescents, also in line with national dental caries statistics.

## Ethnicity

The common practice of adding sugar to bottle-feeds among Asian families in the UK was mentioned earlier in this chapter. This trend has been observed in Australia, the Netherlands, Denmark, and Sweden. Not all Asian immigrants are at similar risk: Muslim (English-speaking and non-English-speaking) and non-Muslim non-English-speaking mothers appear to be special risk groups. The Health Education Authority has produced a most useful briefing paper on *Nutrition in minority ethnic groups: Asians and Afro-Caribbeans in the United Kingdom* (Table 7.5). Since Muslim mothers will not introduce savoury weaning foods that contain non-halal meat and vegetarian households avoid varieties containing meat altogether, there is a tendency to rely heavily on sweet dessert-type baby foods which are often low in protein and iron.

## Schools

Schools vary considerably in their attitude to nutrition and diet. Many schools have excellent policies providing nutritious, attractive meals and restricting snacking within schools. Three epidemiological studies have recorded higher caries experience in children attending schools which sold sweets compared with children in schools which restricted the sale of sweets. Schools often face considerable financial barriers to instilling good dietary practices—schools are often tempted by soft-drink vendors prepared to install vending machines on favourable terms and to sponsor school sports teams, and by the sugar and sugar-related industries who provide teaching material free for schools.

Peer group pressure has a considerable influence on eating habits of children, especially adolescents, both in school and after school. This is enhanced by the preponderance of children bringing packed lunches to school, providing an opportunity to display preferences.

## The role of doctors, dentists, dietitians, and health educators in giving dietary advice for oral health

Contradictory advice rapidly destroys credibility and the consumer's interest in health messages. It is very important that professionals in each country agree about what messages should be given. Regular meetings between sister professional societies is sensible and there are good examples of this occurring. These discussions help to ensure uniformity of advice and reassessment when necessary. The

Table 7.5.
Summary of regional diets of the main Asian groups in Britain by country of origin

| | Indian Punjab | | Gujarat | | Pakistan | Bangladesh |
|---|---|---|---|---|---|---|
| | Sikhs | Hindus | Hindus | Muslims | Muslims | Muslims |
| Main staple cereal | Chapattis | Chapattis | Chapattis or rice | Chapattis or rice | Chapattis | Rice |
| Main fats | Ghee | Ghee | Groundnut or mustard oil; some ghee | Groundnut or mustard oil; some ghee | Ghee or groundnut oil | Groundnut or mustard oil; a little ghee |
| Meat and fish | No beef Some vegetarians; others eat mainly chicken or mutton | No beef Mostly vegetarians | No beef Mostly vegetarians | No pork Halal meat only (usually chicken or mutton) | No pork Halal meat only (usually chicken or mutton) | No pork Halal meat only (usually chicken or mutton) |
| | No fish | No fish | Some fish | Little if any fish | Little fish | A lot of fresh or dried fish |
| Eggs | Not a major part of the diet | Not eaten by strict vegetarians | Not eaten by strict vegetarians | Usually hard boiled, fried, or omelette | Usually hard boiled, fried, or omelette | Few—usually hard boiled, fried, or omelette (in curries) |
| Dairy products | Very important: Milk Yoghurt Curd Cheese | Very important: Milk Yoghurt Curd Cheese | Important: Milk Yoghurt | Fairly important: Milk Yoghurt | Fairly important: Milk Yoghurt | Few: Milk |
| Pulses | Major source of protein | Major source of protein | Major source of protein | Important | Important | Important |
| Vegetables and fruit | Curries Occasional salad Fresh fruit | Curries Occasional salad Fresh fruit | Curries Occasional salad Fresh fruit | Curries Occasional salad Fresh fruit | Curries Occasional salad Fresh fruit | Curries Occasional salad Fresh fruit |

Health Education Authority (1991).

Health Education Authority plays a key role in informing professionals of agreed policies in dietary advice, for example through their excellent policy document *The scientific basis of dental health education*, now in its fourth edition (Box 7.16).

In the USA, the importance of ensuring that paediatricians are adequately informed for their valuable role in the prevention of dental disease has been emphasized: the prescription of fluoride dietary supplements is an area in which close cooperation is required to ensure that dosage schedules are correct for each community.

Box 7.16 **Summary of 'The scientific basis of dental health education'**

1. Diet: reduce the consumption and especially the frequency of intake of sugar-containing food and drink.
2. Tooth-brushing: clean the teeth thoroughly twice every day with a fluoride toothpaste.
3. Fluoridation: request your local water company to supply water with the optimum fluoride level.
4. Dental attendance: have an oral examination every year.

Health Education Authority (1996).

# Summary

- The greatest threat to the dental health of children comes from excessive use of non-milk extrinsic sugars. At present, in children in the UK, these sugars provide about 17 per cent of energy, whereas this figure should be between 0 and 11 per cent for this population.

- Confectionery, soft drinks, biscuits, cakes, and table sugar provide over 80 per cent of non-milk extrinsic sugars in children and are thus the main targets for dietary advice.

- Of particular concern in the infant and young child is the addition of sugar to milk feeds and the frequent and prolonged use of sugary drinks, often used as comforters.

- There are strong social class and ethnic trends in their use.

- Many factors influence food choice, and the necessity to consider these when giving advice, or planning health promotion programmes, will be discussed further in Chapters 9 and 10.

- Malnutrition in pregnancy, neonatally, and in infancy are causes of enamel hypoplasia and, very possibly, increased risk of dental caries.

- Fluoride has a well proven role in the prevention of dental caries, and sensible use of fluoride should actively be encouraged. The best dietary vehicle for fluoride is water. In the absence of water fluoridation, fluoridated salt, milk, or drops and tablets can be considered. In addition to these systemic methods of fluoride administration, children under 6 years of age should have their teeth brushed by their carer with a low-fluoride toothpaste.

- The sensible use of fluorides and the control of consumption of non-milk extrinsic sugars can do much to optimize the oral and dental health of children.

- Erosion of teeth is perceived as a growing problem, especially in adolescents. Soft drinks are likely to be the major dietary cause.

- Sick children sometimes require special diets: dentists should discuss the care of such patients with their medical and dietetic colleagues.

- Correct nutrition plays a key role in ensuring dental health for children. Many different professional groups can each help to ensure that this is achieved.

## Further reading

Department of Health and Social Security (1988). *Present day practice in infant feeding: third report*. Report on health and social subjects, 32. HMSO, London.

Department of Health (1989). *Dietary sugars and human disease*. Report on health and social subjects, 37. HMSO, London.

Department of Health (1994). *Weaning and the weaning diet*. Report on health and social subjects, 45. HMSO, London.

Health Education Authority (1995). *Diet and health in school age children. A briefing paper*. HEA, London.

Ministry of Agriculture, Fisheries and Food (1997). *Healthy diets for infants and young children. A guide for health professionals*. MAFF, London.

Rugg-Gunn, A. J. (1988). *Nutrition and dental health*, Chapter 14. Oxford University Press, Oxford.

# 8

# Nutrition, diet, and oral health of adults

# Nutrition, diet, and oral health of adults

## Introduction

The previous chapter described nutritional guidelines for the UK and what changes in the eating habits of people in this country are necessary to move towards these goals. This information is relevant more widely than just the UK, as many industrialized countries have diets similar to ours and recommendations by authorities in other countries and by the WHO for the world population are compatible with recommendations for the UK.

Chapters 2 to 6 have demonstrated that many oral diseases are diet related and that dietary advice should be an integral part of the oral care of adults. The main aim of this chapter is to draw information given in these early chapters together, so that it is clear what advice you should give to adults attending your practice to help them improve and preserve their oral health. This advice has to be compatible with advice for general health, and the first part of this chapter will review what this general advice should be. Dental staff are in a privileged position, compared with many health care groups, in that they see a large proportion of the population regularly, usually at least once a year. They have, therefore, a very valuable role in promoting good eating habits in the general population. This is recognized by government who try to ensure that dentists, along with other health professionals, are adequately trained in nutrition.

## Advice for general health in adults

The previous chapter emphasized that the broad guidelines for healthy eating were now well established. The 1991 Department of Health COMA report *Dietary reference values for food, energy and nutrients for the United Kingdom* was an important, authoritative statement on nutritional targets (Table 8.1).

Presently, we get too little of our energy from complex carbohydrates (starches) and too much from fat and non-milk extrinsic sugars. This very much applies to adults. The results of a survey of UK adults, 16–64 years of age, are given in Table 8.2 and indicate, when compared with Table 8.1, how much diet must change in the UK.

Two other Department of Health COMA reports are relevant to this discussion. First, *The nutrition of elderly people* published in 1992. This contains 21 recommendations for maintaining good nutritional status in the elderly—seven of these are given in Box 8.1. As exercise decreases with age, food energy intake also decreases. Requirements for nutrients do not necessarily decrease with food energy requirements, which means that the nutrient density of diets for elderly people should be high. Part of the reason for recommending that non-milk extrinsic sugars should be no more than 10 per cent of food energy in this group

Table 8.1.

Dietary reference values for fat and carbohydrate for adults as a percentage of daily total energy intake (percentage of food energy)

| | Population average |
|---|---|
| Saturated fatty acids (maximum) | 10 (11) |
| Total fat (maximum) | 33 (35) |
| Non-milk extrinsic sugars (maximum) | 10 (11) |
| Intrinsic and milk sugars and starch (minimum) | 37 (39) |
| Total carbohydrate | 47 (50) |
| Non-starch polysaccharide (g/day) | 18 |

Figures in parentheses apply when alcohol consumption is excluded. Source: Department of Health (1991).

Table 8.2.

Daily nutritional intake of UK adults aged 16–64 years, surveyed in 1987

| | Men | Women |
|---|---|---|
| Number | 1087 | 1110 |
| Energy (MJ) | 10.3 | 7.1 |
| Fat[a] | 40.4% | 40.3% |
| Carbohydrate[a] | 44.7% | 44.2% |
| Starch[a] | 25.8% | 24.5% |
| Sugars[a] | 18.9% | 19.7% |

[a] As % energy from food. Office of Population Censuses and Surveys (1990).

is to ensure that consumption of sugary foods does not blunt the nutritional density of the diet. The report recognizes, however, that the main reason for restricting consumption of non-milk extrinsic sugars is to control dental caries in this group of people, who are now much more likely to have their own teeth than was the case in the past.

The report sounded a warning about being overzealous in restricting sugar intake for all elderly people. Paragraph 6.1.4 in the report says:

There may however be individual circumstances where appropriate intakes of simple sugars may be higher than the recommendations for the elderly population as a whole. Very elderly people, especially during episodes of ill health, may find difficulty in consuming sufficient dietary energy given that alter-

## Box 8.1 Some recommendations from the COMA report on nutrition of elderly people

- The recommendations of the Panel on Dietary Reference Values of the Committee on Medical Aspects of Food Policy are endorsed. The working party recommends that elderly people should reduce dietary intakes of fat and simple sugars and increase intakes of starchy foods, non-starch polysaccharides, and vitamin D.
- Elderly people should derive their dietary intakes from a diet containing a variety of nutrient-dense foods.
- For the majority of elderly people, the same recommendations concerning the dietary intake of non-milk extrinsic sugars apply as for the younger adult population.
- Intakes of non-starch polysaccharides comparable to those recommended for the general population are advised for most elderly people. Foods with high phytate content, especially raw bran, should be avoided or used sparingly.
- Elderly people, in common with those of all ages, should be advised to eat more fresh vegetables, fruit, and whole grain cereals.
- The Working Group endorsed the WHO recommendations that 6 g/day sodium chloride would be a reasonable average intake for the elderly population in the UK, and recommends that the present average dietary salt intakes should be reduced to meet this level.
- Health professionals should be made aware of the impact of nutritional status on the development of and recovery from illness.

native energy sources such as fat may be less desirable or starchy foods may be difficult to consume. Sugar not only contains energy itself but may also help to increase the palatability to sick people and so encourage more food to be eaten.

Strokes are relatively common in elderly people and since blood pressure and salt consumption are positively related, the report recommends (with some caution) that salt intake for most elderly people should be reduced.

Overall, it can be seen that advice for the elderly is pretty similar to advice for other adults—increase consumption of staple starchy foods, fresh fruit, and vegetables. These are often difficult foods to bite and chew and this important subject will be returned to later in this chapter. Many of these more desirable foods need more preparation, which some elderly people find difficult. Finally, for a variety of reasons, including the interactions of some drugs which may be taken by elderly people, absorption of nutrients from the alimentary canal may be reduced in this group.

Two Department of Health reports on specific diseases of adulthood are relevant: *Nutritional aspects of cardiovascular disease* published in 1994 (Box 8.2) and *Nutritional aspects of the development of cancer* published in 1998 (Box 8.3). Both of these re-emphasize the message of the important protective effect of vegetables, fruit, and complex carbohydrates.

## Box 8.2 Some recommendations from the COMA report on nutrition and cardiovascular disease

- Maintain a desirable weight (body mass index between 20 and 25).
- The contribution of dietary fat to dietary energy should be reduced to about 35 per cent, with the contribution of saturated fatty acids no more than 10 per cent of dietary energy intake.
- Eat at least two portions of fish per week, one of which should be oily fish.
- Consumption of vegetables, fruit, potatoes, and bread should increase by at least 50 per cent.

Box 8.3 **Some recommendations from the COMA report on nutritional aspects of cancer**

- Maintain a healthy body weight (body mass index within the range 20–25) and do not increase it during adult life.

- Increase intakes of a wide variety of fruits and vegetables.

- Increase intakes of non-starch polysaccharides (dietary fibre) from a variety of food sources.

- For adults, individuals' consumption of red and processed meat should not rise; higher consumers should consider a reduction; and as a consequence of this the population average will fall.

- These recommendations should be followed in the context of COMA's wider recommendations for a balanced diet rich in cereals, fruits, and vegetables.

Box 8.4 **Eight guidelines for a healthy diet: a guide for nutrition education**

1. Enjoy your food.
2. Eat a variety of different foods.
3. Eat the right amount to be a healthy weight.
4. Eat plenty of foods rich in starch and fibre.
5. Eat plenty of fruit and vegetables.
6. Don't eat too many foods that contain a lot of fat.
7. Don't have sugary foods and drinks too often.
8. If you drink alcohol, drink sensibly.

Health Education Authority (1997).

You will need to give advice to your patients in terms of foods; a very useful document in this regard is *Eight guidelines for a healthy diet* published by the Health Education Authority in 1997. These eight guidelines are given in Box 8.4. The rest of this chapter will examine what advice, compatible with advice for maintaining general health, is appropriate, first for adults and then for elderly people (those aged 65 years and over), for maintaining oral health.

## Oral diseases in adults

The dental state of adults in the UK is changing fast. In 1968, over one third of adults over the age of 16 years had no natural teeth at all. By 1988, the proportion of edentulous people had fallen to 21 per cent (Table 8.3). From the results of the national surveys in 1968, 1978, and 1988, it is possible to predict the dental state of adults in 30 years time. You can see that the proportion of edentulous adults is expected to fall to 6 per cent of all adults, and four out of five of those aged 75 years and over will retain at least some of their teeth, by 2038.

The 1988 UK Adult Dental Health survey took the presence of 21 teeth in the mouth as an indication of a functional natural dentition. While 77 per cent

Table 8.3.
**Total tooth loss in UK adults, recorded in 1968–88 and predicted up to 2038**

| Year | 1968 | 1978 | 1988 | 1998 | 2008 | 2018 | 2028 | 2038 |
|---|---|---|---|---|---|---|---|---|
| All adults (%) | 37 | 30 | 21 | 14 | 10 | 7 | 6 | 6 |
| 75+ years (%) | 88 | 79 | 80 | 64 | 48 | 34 | 23 | 19 |

Office of Population Censuses and Surveys (1990).

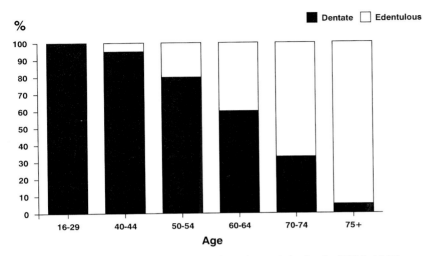

**Figure 8.1** Proportion of dentate and edentulous adults in the UK in 1988, according to age. Source: Office of Population Censuses and Surveys (1990).

of adults aged 16–64 years had 21 or more natural teeth, this is expected to rise to 95 per cent by 2018 (Table 8.4). Thus, adults are expected to keep more of their own teeth for longer. This has two implications: first, food choice is less likely to be affected by impaired dentitions in the future with the prospect of improving general health and, second, that there will be more teeth to protect from dental decay and dental erosion. There is no doubt that teeth do decay in adulthood and, in 1988, the average number of decayed, missing, and filled teeth (DMFT) for dentate adults was 17, leaving 15 sound teeth out of a total of 32

Table 8.4

Percentage of adults in the UK who had in 1988 and are predicted to have in 1998, 2008, and 2018, 21 or more natural teeth

| Age (years) | 1988 | 1998 | 2008 | 2018 |
|---|---|---|---|---|
| 16–24 | 100 | 100 | 100 | 100 |
| 25–34 | 95 | 98 | 98 | 98 |
| 35–44 | 83 | 93 | 96 | 96 |
| 45–54 | 60 | 78 | 88 | 91 |
| 55–64 | 30 | 56 | 74 | 84 |
| 16–64 | 77 | 87 | 92 | 95 |

Office of Population Censuses and Surveys (1990).

Table 8.5.
Mean number of teeth affected by disease in dentate adults
in the UK in 1988

| Average number of teeth | | | |
|---|---|---|---|
| Missing | 7.8 | | |
| Decayed | 1.0 | 9.4 | 17.2 |
| Filled | 8.4 | | |
| Sound | 14.8 | | |
| % with crowns | 26 | | |
| % with exposed roots | 67 | | |
| Average number of decayed or filled roots | 0.7 | | |

Office of Population Censuses and Surveys (1990).

teeth (Table 8.5). The 1995 National Diet and Nutrition Survey showed, yet again, the link between consumption of non-milk extrinsic sugars and root caries in elderly people.

The social costs of dental ill health in adults are considerable. In the USA, over 100 million hours are lost from work for dental reasons, with a quarter of the population reporting work-loss related to dental treatment per year. Dental disease has been shown to have a negative impact on psychological well-being and there is considerable potential for improving older people's psychological well-being and quality of life by improving oral health. It should be noted that dental health is not perceived by older people as being related to general health; dental health behaviour is considered part of personal routine behaviour and attendance at a dentist currently tends to be perceived as a purely problem-solving exercise. Disease-preventive activities, including dietary advice, which are valued by the patient, are a way of trying to encourage adults to seek regular attendance and so maximize the opportunity to preserve their dentition. Regular attendance provides an opportunity to screen for other diet-related diseases of the hard and soft oral tissues, as discussed in Chapter 5.

# Dietary advice for the preservation of the dentition in adult life

## The importance of preserving a functional dentition

People wish to retain their teeth for a variety of reasons—aesthetics, function, the feeling that teeth are part of the body, and the perceived inferiority of the artificial substitutes. But, since quality of food choice and nutrient intake are compromised by a poor dentition, dentists should encourage and assist the retention of functional, natural teeth. You need to tell patients of the nutritional impact that loss of occluding pairs of teeth may have. If fixed or removable prostheses are provided, it is very important to give dietary advice to the patient.

## Sugar and dental caries

Dental caries is still the biggest threat to teeth in the adult. The dietary cause of caries is quite clear and was discussed in Chapter 3. As the Health Education Authority's booklet *The scientific basis of dental health education* says, 'reduce the consumption and especially the frequency of intake of sugar-containing food and drink'. This is as applicable to adults as it is to children. Caries of the roots of teeth occurs in adults (Fig. 8.2). The aetiology of root caries is broadly similar to coronal caries, so that dietary advice for the prevention of root caries is essentially the same as for the prevention of coronal caries.

Advice, therefore, should be directed towards reducing both the amount of sugars consumed and the frequency of consumption of sugars. In practice, amount and frequency are likely to be closely correlated so that reduction in one is likely to lead to a reduction in the other.

Lifestyle affects eating habits considerably. People at work may have less opportunity to snack than people at home. Results of surveys of adult dental health have revealed higher dental disease experience in women than men, but this may well be a reflection of different attitudes to tooth preservation rather than different eating habits. There is anecdotal evidence of substantial caries development occurring in men on retirement from work, with the suggestion that this is due to an increase in snacking caused by more spare time. For many older people, the warmest room in the house is often the kitchen, which encourages frequent eating in cold climates. Social contacts for older people often involve tea and biscuits. While such social contacts are very desirable for improving quality of life, the dietary implications of such habits may need to be examined closely in a small proportion of people. Adults over the age of 60–65 years obtain more of their energy from non-milk extrinsic sugars than do those under 60–65 years of age. There is a strong trend towards a higher level of purchase of packaged sugar by older 'housewives' than by younger 'housewives'.

The dental advantages of the use of non-sugar sweeteners were also discussed in Chapter 3. As people retain their natural teeth for longer, so the relevance of non-sugar sweeteners increases. For children, priority foods for sugar substitution were confectionery, soft drinks, table sugar, and medicines. This list also seems appropriate for adults. Tea, coffee, and other hot drinks may be relatively more popular than soft drinks in adults and the use of non-sugar sweeteners in place of sugar in these drinks could be of considerable benefit, especially as many of these older adults have been in the habit of sweetening their hot drinks all their lives. We will discuss the important subject of medicines later in this chapter.

## Dental erosion

Chapter 4 described how dental erosion can be caused by intrinsic and extrinsic factors. In children, the extrinsic factors are likely to be more important on a population basis, with soft drinks seen as the main culprit. In adults, intrinsic causes may be relatively more important than in children. Regurgitation of gastric contents is strongly related to excessive alcohol consumption, which is all too prevalent in adulthood. Intestinal pathologies in later life are a further cause of regurgitation and therefore erosion. The very young and the very elderly are

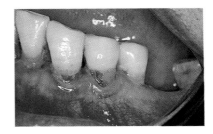

**Figure 8.2** Caries affecting the root surfaces of these mandibular teeth. Reproduced with permission of Dr J Steele.

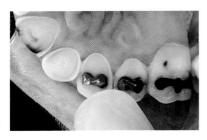

**Figure 8.3** Severe dental erosion affecting the palatal surfaces of the maxillary teeth particularly, in a patient consuming three cans of a cola beverage per day. Reproduced with permission of Dr S Jones.

two groups likely to be prescribed liquid oral medicines rather than tablets. Liquid oral medicines are, therefore, a potential cause of erosion for elderly people where medication is common (see below).

Fresh fruit, fruit juices, and pickled vegetables are recognized causes of dental erosion in adults. There is, therefore, a potential conflict in advice for general and dental health. We should encourage the population to increase consumption of fresh fruit and vegetables and yet recognize that some dental erosion is a price that will have to be paid. It would not be right for dentists to advise against consumption of these highly desirable food groups. However, there are some fruit-eating habits which we can advise against without impairing good dietary goals. Some people get pleasure from sucking citrus fruit, leaving it in their mouth, often between their teeth, for long periods. This has no nutritional advantage and is very erosive. Likewise holding fruit juices in the mouth is potentially erosive and should be advised against. In cases where erosion from fruit juices is a potential problem, a drinking straw is useful for depositing the juice towards the back of the mouth. The patient should, however, be counselled that this may transfer the impact of drinking potentially erosive drinks from the teeth at the front of the mouth to the molars (Fig. 8.3).

## Dietary fluoride and prevention of dental disease

The very important role of fluoride in the prevention of dental caries was discussed in Chapters 2 and 3. Adjustment of the concentration of fluoride in drinking water to the optimum for that community has been implemented worldwide—in at least 39 countries reaching at least 210 million people—and is effective—reducing caries experience by about half on average. Most studies have investigated the effectiveness of fluoride in children, since it is easier to identify and examine lifelong residents of a young age in fluoridated and fluoride-deficient communities. Nevertheless, there have been several surveys which have shown that the dental health of adults is considerably better when they have lived in communities with optimum amounts of fluoride in drinking water. This applies to both coronal and root surface caries, an observation which highlights the common aetiology of these two types of lesions.

As far as can be seen, there are no reports of the caries-preventive effect of other forms of dietary fluoride—tablets, salt, or milk—in adults, but it must be appreciated that these have been used on a public health basis only comparatively recently and investigated much less comprehensively, compared with water fluoridation. Fluoride has been used topically (locally in the mouth) to prevent dental caries in adults with considerable success. The effect of fluoride on resorption of alveolar bone and periodontal disease will be considered in the next section.

## Nutrition and periodontal disease

The main conclusion from the review of this subject in Chapter 5 was that there is little evidence that nutritional deficiencies affect the occurrence or progression of periodontal disease in humans. The overriding factor in the cause, prevention, and treatment of periodontal disease and its precursor, gingivitis, is control of dental plaque. Overall, periodontal tissues will benefit when nutrition is adequate but dietary supplementation above what is commonly accepted as adequate levels does not seem to improve periodontal health further. Evidence is emerging that folate mouth-rinses may be beneficial in the control of gingivitis in circumstances where the gingival tissues may be folate-deficient (e.g. in pregnancy or phenytoin therapy) but widespread prescription of folate for the prevention and control of gingivitis is premature.

Scurvy is the only deficiency disease in which the periodontal tissues are primarily affected. It is now rare, but should be suspected in patients with a tender mouth or bleeding swollen gums: elderly men living on their own seem to be at greatest risk. Regression of the disease rapidly follows vitamin C therapy.

The alveolar bone is important in supporting teeth when they are present and for supporting dentures after teeth are lost. Calcium and vitamin D deficiencies have been shown in animal experiments to accelerate periodontal destruction but there is much less evidence in humans. Where deficiencies exist, dietary advice to restore intake to adequate levels is sensible, as this will benefit the skeleton in general, including dental alveolar bone. Supplementation when the diet is already adequate is not warranted.

Some studies have reported less periodontal destruction in residents of communities with adequate levels of fluoride in drinking water supplies than in residents of low-fluoride areas. Fluoride has been used in treatment of general osteoporosis, although its effectiveness is not universally accepted.

# Advice for elderly people

A large number of factors influence food choice in elderly people and these must be considered when advising on nutrition for general and oral health. These are listed in Table 8.6. Fresh fruit and vegetables are often considered expensive, certainly in relation to the food energy provided; they are heavy to carry, and vegetables usually require preparation and cooking. They are also more perishable than many other foods. Not only may cooking facilities be poor in some older peoples' homes but the ability and will to prepare food and cook it may have diminished. There is concern in many countries about the quality of diets provided for elderly people who live in institutions; even some hospitals are not immune to this criticism. Old age brings many changes in physiological function—in taste, smell, and gastrointestinal functions. Elderly people are more likely than other people to be on drugs which interfere with absorption and utilization of nutrients. The effects of a poor dentition and poor salivary flow will now be considered in more detail.

The value of teeth in nutrition was considered in Chapter 6. The general conclusions were that lack of natural teeth affects ability to chew and food choice. There was less direct evidence that nutrition was affected, although consumption of non-starch polysaccharides is low in those with impaired dentitions. Reduced energy intake and iron (from meats), vitamin C, and calcium were seen as other risk nutrients in elderly people. There is very little direct evidence that an impaired dentition affects general health but this could be due to the difficulty in mounting the required comprehensive longitudinal studies. It is reasonable to assume that if consumption of fruits and vegetables is reduced because of poor teeth, general health is at increased risk.

Table 8.6.
Some factors influencing food intake and nutrition in older people

| Factor | Effect |
|---|---|
| Economic | Choice of foods |
| | Cooking facilities |
| | Transport to shops |
| Social | Living alone |
| | Housebound |
| | Bereavement |
| Psychosocial—patient behaviour | Senility |
| | Depression |
| | Psychosis |
| | Unadaptability |
| | Alcohol consumption |
| Psychosocial—society behaviour | Retirement and nursing homes |
| | Home helps |
| Physiological and pathological | Changes in gastrointestinal function |
| | Impaired taste and smell |
| | Impaired function of heart, lungs, and kidneys |
| | Arthritis and immobility |
| | Diabetes mellitus |
| | Poor dentition |
| | Hyposalivation |
| Interaction of drugs with nutrients | Changes in absorption |
| | Changes in metabolism |

The hazard of choking on food in elderly people was also discussed in Chapter 6. There are probably several reasons for the increased risk:

- A poor dentition may make it harder for foods to be broken down to a small size suitable for swallowing.
- Lack of saliva will make bolus formation more difficult.
- Dentures covering the oral mucosa reduce the feedback on food size and its condition.
- Swallowing may be impaired in elderly people due to stroke or other illnesses.

Elderly patients therefore need to be advised of the importance of cutting up food before putting it in the mouth and for taking time to chew foods before swallowing.

The importance of saliva has been highlighted several times already. The general functions of saliva are summarized in Table 8.7. Saliva is the principal protector of the hard and soft tissues. When salivary flow is diminished, eating is less enjoyable and can be uncomfortable; swallowing a bolus of food can be difficult. Salivary flow rate is thought to decrease with age but this is not a simple relationship. Flow rate is virtually undiminished in healthy elderly people, but is lower in those who are not in good health. About 20 per cent of people up to 50 years of age and 40 per cent of elderly people complain of a dry mouth.

The first sign of hyposalivation or xerostomia (dry mouth) is often an unexpected increase in dental caries. Other symptoms include the need to drink water; difficulty with speech, eating, and swallowing; difficulty with dentures; cracking at the corners of the mouth; a burning sensation on the tongue associated with fissuring of the tongue; and alteration of taste. Measurement of salivary flow is easy in theory but in practice needs considerable care, since psychic factors (e.g. apprehension, degree of lighting) can influence considerably the amount of saliva collected. Measurement of total salivary flow is generally useful, although recording flow from one gland is feasible and necessary in some circumstances.

Hypofunction of the salivary glands is caused by a number of diseases or conditions, the most important being drugs, irradiation, organic diseases, psychological disorders, and decreased chewing. These often occur in elderly people so it is not surprising that hyposalivation is prevalent in these age groups. A large number of drugs cause salivary hypofunction, as can be seen in Box 8.5. Usually these drugs do not permanently damage the glands and salivary flow returns to

## Table 8.7.
### The general functions of saliva

| Digestive functions | Protective functions |
| --- | --- |
| Assisting the mastication of food | Ensuring comfort through lubrication |
| Forming a bolus | Preventing desiccation of oral mucosa, gingivae, and lips |
| Assisting in swallowing of bolus | Antimicrobial: |
| Metabolism of starch | lavage |
| | bacteriostatic, bactericidal |
| | inhibiting adhesion of bacteria |
| | aggregation of bacteria |
| | Buffering: |
| | within saliva |
| | within dental plaque |
| | Removal of toxins (including carcinogens) |
| | Taste perception |
| | Aids speech |

## Box 8.5 Drugs causing xerostomia

- Anxiolytics
- Antidepressants
- Tricyclic antidepressants
- Monoamine oxidase inhibitors
- Hypnotics
- Antipsychotics
- Antimanics
- Antiparkinsonian drugs
- Some asthma inhalers
- Bronchodilators
- Antihistamines
- Decongestants
- Ganglion-blocking agents

It is important to check the *British National Formulary* regularly to add to or modify this list.

near normal if the drug therapy is stopped. Salivary glands are sensitive to irradiation and severe irreversible hypofunction follows significant irradiation used to treat oral neoplasms. Destruction of the salivary gland tissues is a feature of many autoimmune diseases, including Sjögren's syndrome and rheumatoid arthritis. Depression and anxiety may contribute to hyposalivation which is often compounded by the powerful xerostomic effect of tricyclic antidepressant drugs used to treat these disorders. Disuse atrophy affects the salivary glands as it does other tissues.

While disease can cause atrophy, chewing can increase the size of salivary glands and increase salivary flow. Thus, recommending foods which require chewing is likely to improve oral health, not only by causing a strong flow of saliva while food is chewed but also improving the ability of glands to respond to future stimuli. This is an important reason for recommending chewing sugarless gum.

People suffering from hyposalivation or xerostomia tend to sip liquids to alleviate their discomfort. Milk can be recommended as a salivary substitute. Types of artificial saliva, apart from milk, fall into three groups—glycerine and lemon, those based on carboxymethylcellulose, and those based on mucin. Glycerine and lemon is the simplest but, if natural teeth are present, is potentially erosive. In addition, glycerine is astringent and may 'sting' the soft tissues. Mucin-based artificial salivas have the best properties and are commercially available in many countries. Artificial saliva is usually taken from a small cup as a mouthwash (Fig. 8.4) or as a spray. Some saliva substitutes are based on pig products and are thus contraindicated in vegetarians and people of some religions.

The use of medication increases in older people, with polypharmacy common among the elderly. About 40 per cent of elderly people take at least one medication daily and persons over the age of 70 years are reported to receive an average of 20 prescriptions yearly. As has been mentioned already, this has two effects:

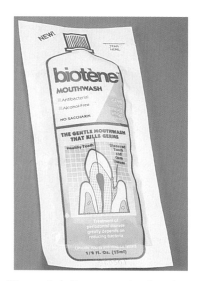

**Figure 8.4** One example of a saliva substitute which is available also as a spray and a toothpaste for use at different times during the day.

Table 8.8.
## Management of xerostomia

| Signs and symptoms | Management |
|---|---|
| Dry mouth | Improve oral hygiene/saliva substitutes |
| Difficulty with speech | Chlorhexidine gel or mouth-rinse |
| Difficulty with swallowing | Avoid sugar-sweetened drinks/confectionery |
| Difficulty with dentures | Frequent sips of iced water |
| Disturbed taste sensation | Suck chips of ice |
| Increased caries rate | Evian atomized spray |
| Increased periodontal disease | Fluoride mouth-rinse, chlorhexidine mouth-rinse |
| Oral infections | Prescribe as appropriate |
| Salivary gland infections | Refer for opinion |

first, many drugs depress salivary secretion, increasing the risk of oral disease and, second, some medicines contain sugar, particularly the liquid oral medicines which some elderly people prefer. This highlights the importance of obtaining a full medical history, including drug-taking, from patients. You should not seek to change medication without the approval of the prescriber, but there may be opportunities to advise the patient to ask for (if on prescription) or choose (if being bought over the counter) a sugar-free alternative.

In Chapter 5, it was suggested that the mouth was the mirror of the body. Many systemic illnesses give rise to oral signs, and chief among these are nutritional deficiency diseases. The dental practitioner is very well placed to recognize these lesions, advise the patient, and refer the patient for further care if necessary. This underlines the importance of full examination of the oral mucosa, lips, and perioral tissues.

Another reason for the thorough and systematic examination of the oral mucosa is that the dental practitioner may be the first to observe and recognize oral cancers or their pre-malignant precursors. The dietary messages regarding the prevention of oral cancers are quite clear—avoid excessive alcohol consumption (and smoking) and eat fresh fruit and vegetables. As far as effectiveness of change is concerned, reducing smoking and alcohol consumption is more effective than increasing fruit and vegetable consumption.

Dental practitioners, as part of the broader health team, should take the appropriate opportunities to convey these important health promotion messages. However, there is much more to changing eating habits of adults, particularly the elderly, than just giving advice—these aspects will be considered in Chapter 10.

## Summary

- Current recommendations for nutritional intake in adults in the UK, which are in agreement with international guidelines and recommendations in several other developed countries, call for a reduction in intake of dietary fats and non-milk extrinsic sugars and an increase in intake of starchy foods, fresh fruit, and vegetables. If implemented, substantial improvements in dental and general health can be expected in the population.

- Older adults are keeping more of their teeth for longer.

- Dental caries is still a major oral disease in adults. Consumption of non-milk extrinsic sugars seems to be higher in older adults than in younger adults, and should be decreased.

- Salivary flow does not diminish appreciably with age in the healthy person. However, salivary flow is lower in older people with poor health compared with older people in good health so that, overall, the mean population salivary flow is lower in the elderly population. There is a wide variety of causes of hyposalivation, one of the most important being medication.

- A tendency towards reduced salivary flow, together with a higher sugar intake and increased gingival recession, places the dentate older person at greater risk of dental caries (coronal and root caries) than other adults.

**Box 8.6 Commercial saliva substitutes**

- \* Glandosane (Fresenius)—denture wearers only; pH is low enough to cause erosion

- \* Saliva Orthana (Nycomed)—porcine derivatives unsuitable for some ethnic groups and vegetarians

- ◊ Luborant (Antigen)—contains lactose peroxidase which increases oral defence mechanisms; viscosity increases as temperature increases; contains fluoride

- • Oral balance/Biotene (Laclede UK)—available as mouth-rinse, lozenges, and toothpaste for sustained effect.

---

- \* Approved for use in patients with dry mouth as a result of radiotherapy or sicca syndrome

- ◊ licensed for any condition

- • Not in BNF but available on NHS prescription.

- Lifestyles are likely to change upon retirement from work, possibly leading to more opportunity to snack. Common snacks are likely to be sugared tea and biscuits. Social contacts are important for the well-being of older people, but the threat to dental health of dentate persons of frequent snacking habits is apparent.

- Consumption of medicines increases with age. The threat to the teeth of dentate people taking sugar-containing medicines daily, long term should be recognized and sugar-free formulations chosen. Attention should be given to both prescription medicines and over-the-counter sales.

- In contrast to dental caries, periodontal disease is little influenced by nutrition or dietary habits. Plaque removal with a toothbrush is much more important.

- Ingestion of an optimum level of fluoride from the water supply (around 1 mg F/l in temperate climates) throughout life significantly reduces dental caries experience in adults; some benefit to periodontal health may also occur.

- The most important causes of dental erosion in adults are excessive regurgitation, fruit and pickled vegetable consumption, and acidic drinks. Dental erosion is becoming a public health issue and is certainly a severe problem in some patients.

- The adverse effect that loss of teeth has on food choice and nutrient intake should be explained to patients: preservation of a functional, natural dentition is desirable. Dietary advice must accompany the provision of fixed or removable prostheses.

- Dental practitioners are in an excellent position to examine the oral mucosa for signs of systemic disease and oral malignancies. They should be prepared to give broad advice for the prevention of these diseases.

## Further reading

Billings, R. J., Proskin, H. M., and Moss, M. E. (1996). Xerostomia and associated factors in a community-dwelling adult population. *Community Dent. Oral Epidemiol.* 24, 312–16.

Department of Health (1991). *Dietary reference values for food energy and nutrients for the United Kingdom*. Report on health and social subjects, 41. HMSO, London.

Department of Health (1992). *The nutrition of elderly people*. Report on health and social subjects, 43. HMSO, London.

Department of Health (1994) *Nutritional aspects of cardiovascular disease*. Report on health and social subjects, 46. HMSO, London.

Department of Health (1998) *Nutritional aspects of the development of cancer*. Report on health and social subjects, 48. The Stationery Office, London

Johansson, I., Tidehag, P., Lundberg, V., and Hallmans, G. (1994). Dental status, diet and cardiovascular risk factors in middle-aged people in northern Sweden. *Community Dent. Oral Epidemiol.* 22, 431–6.

Rogers, L. and Sharp, I. (eds) (1997). *Preventing coronary heart disease*. National Heart Forum, London.

Rugg-Gunn, A. J. (1993). *Nutrition and dental health*, Chapter 15. Oxford University Press, Oxford.

Steele, J. G., Sheilam, A., Marcenes, W., and Walls, A. W. G. (1998) *National diet and nutrition survey: people aged 65 years and over; Vol. 2, report of the oral health survey*. The Stationery Office, London.

Todd, J. E. and Lader, D. (1991) *Adult dental health 1988 United Kingdom*. Office of population censuses and surveys. HMSO, London.

# 9

# How national and community food policies influence diet

# How national and community food policies influence diet

## Introduction

You still sometimes hear the phrase 'you can't change peoples' diet'. That is not true. Our diet in the UK has changed much—mostly for the better, but in some aspects for the worse. National and community food policies should ensure that it changes for the better and this is the basis for much of public health medicine and public health dentistry. Some of the landmarks of changes in the diet of people in the UK are given in Table 9.1. Children in the UK are taller and healthier than they have ever been and life expectancy has increased steadily. Improvements in housing and sanitation, and in medical immunization and

## Box 9.1 Trends in food consumption in the UK

The National Food Survey (NFS) began in the UK in 1940 and is still going. It is undertaken annually by the Ministry of Agriculture, Fisheries and Food (MAFF) and provides a valuable continuing snapshot of food purchase, and hence consumption, by people in the UK. Data are provided for different regions of the UK, socioeconomic groups, household composition, age of the 'housewife', and seasons. While these data have been most valuable, it should be appreciated that they do refer to food purchase and exclude, until recently, foods eaten outside the home and confectionery. Figure 9.1 shows trends in consumption of major food groups over the past 50 years. The decline in vegetable consumption is very largely due to the fall in consumption of potatoes (by about one third). Bread consumption has fallen by around two thirds. Whole milk consumption has declined markedly; skimmed and semi-skimmed milk consumption has risen but is still, in percentage terms, small. These falls are partly explained by the decrease in energy expenditure due to a more sedentary lifestyle, but are partly offset by the increased consumption of meat and meat products. The effect of these changes on nutrient intake can be seen in Fig. 9.2. The target for fat intake is no more than 35 per cent of energy—as can be seen, it used to be at this figure in the 1940s and early 50s but it is now about 42 per cent.

The NFS gives information on consumption of packaged sugar only. This has declined markedly as home cooking has declined. A better picture of sugar consumption in the UK is obtained from other government statistics which include sugar in manufactured foods. These data are given in Fig. 9.3. Sugar consumption was restricted during the two World Wars and rose to its highest level in the late 1950s, 1960s, and early 1970s. National data on caries prevalence in children parallel these figures quite closely—caries prevalence dipped during and after the two World Wars and reached its highest point in the 1960s and early 1970s.

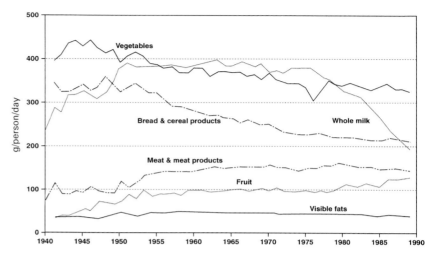

**Figure 9.1** Trends in consumption of major food groups, 1940–90, in Great Britain. Based on Ministry of Agriculture, Fisheries and Food (1991).

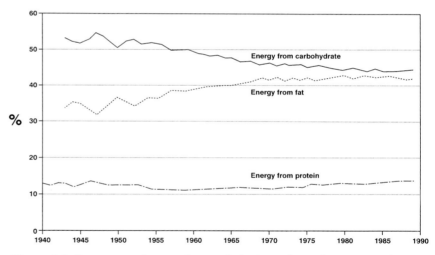

**Figure 9.2** Percentage of energy from carbohydrate, fat, and protein, 1940–90, in Great Britain. Based on Ministry of Agriculture, Fisheries and Food (1991).

treatments have been very important, but improvements in nutrition of the population has been critical too. However, there is definitely no room for complacency: incidences of cardiovascular disease, strokes, and cancer—all having significant dietary components—are high in the UK, substantially higher than in other countries. Obesity is rising and, as it is a risk factor for many diseases, this is of considerable concern. One of the biggest challenges at the present time

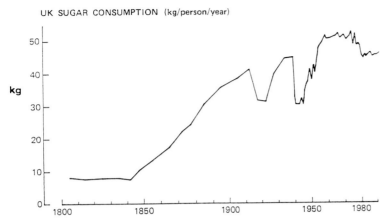

UK SUGAR CONSUMPTION (kg/person/year)

**Figure 9.3** UK Sugar consumption, 1850–1990. Sugar equates to added sugars.

is to understand and successfully manage the rise in the use of convenience foods. On the positive side, supermarkets provide an enormous range of nutritious, well presented foods at prices affordable by the majority of people during vastly extended opening times. On the negative side, the rise in the supermarket has meant that people have to travel further to buy their food and shopping takes longer and may involve carrying heavy bags. The rise in convenience foods has allowed more time for other activities—work or leisure—but has had several adverse effects. Food preparation and cooking at home has declined, resulting in loss of these skills and a shift in control over consumption from the cook at home to the manufacturer of convenience foods. By the mid 1990s, 70 per cent or more of all foods consumed in countries in northern Europe were processed, preserved, and/or packaged in some way.

The effect of these developments should not be underestimated. In northern Europe the consumption of potatoes has fallen and a large proportion of potatoes is now consumed as potato products, for example as chips and crisps, rather than in their fresh state. Processing of potatoes increases their monetary value very substantially but at a cost in nutritional terms of a marked increase in fat consumption.

Similar examples can be given relating to sugar and salt consumption. Sugar intakes have been declining throughout northern Europe when expressed in terms of free sucrose bought in bags as refined sugar. However, the sugar content of food items has increased and new sugar products, such as soft drinks, are an increasingly prominent component of the diet, sustained and promoted by intense advertising. About 70 per cent of sugars consumed are now what can be termed 'added sugars'.

Food manufactures have recognized the usefulness of salt as a taste enhancer so that salt is an important ingredient of commercially produced soups and a variety of manufactured foods, so that now 85 per cent of the population's salt intake comes from non-household sources where the consumer cannot use his or her discretion. New processing techniques improve flavour, and sugars, fats, salt, and spices are added to enhance the texture, crispness, and taste of products.

Table 9.1.
Changes in diet in the UK

| | |
|---|---|
| Before 1850 | Working classes—monotony and too little food. |
| | Upper classes—becoming varied, elaborate, and affordable. |
| 1850–1900 | Growth of food industry (e.g. Liptons, Cadburys and Huntley & Palmer). |
| | Reduction and then removal of tax on sugar imports |
| Early 1900s | National recommendations for infant and childhood feeding; the state taking increasing responsibility for the health of the nation; school meals start. |
| | Rejection of 40% of volunteers for armed forces because of poor physical condition (including poor dental health). |
| 1914–1939 | Emergence of nutrition as a science; the era of discovery of vitamins. |
| | During First World War, diet of the poor actually improved due to full employment; sugar imports decreased. |
| | The depression in the 1930s resulted in concerns as expressed in Boyd Orr's *Food, health and income.* |
| Second World War | Ministry of Food established. |
| | Food rationing: the basis of rationing was physiological requirements and supplements to prevent deficiency diseases. |
| | Sugar availability fell sharply. |
| | Diet improved for some sectors of the population. |
| Post-war years | Food rationing did not finally end until 1954. |
| | Fortification of many foods (e.g. margarine, bread) continued. |
| | Ministry of Agriculture, Fisheries and Food (MAFF) created in 1955. |
| | National Food Survey (NFS) began in 1940; gives picture of purchase of foods. |
| | Emergence of the supermarket. |
| | Decline in work canteens and school meals. |
| | 'Market forces' given free rein. |
| | The 'farming revolution' increasing productivity. |
| | Refrigerators and freezers common. |
| | Variety and availability of foods increases enormously. |
| | Decline in teaching of cooking skills. |
| | Increase in both parents working outside the home. |
| | Rise in use of convenience foods. |
| | Deficiency diseases rare. |
| | Physical activity decreases; obesity increases. |
| | Formation of Food Standards Agency in 1998. |

Based on James (1993)

Thus, wherever the food industry is a major source of food products, there has been a natural tendency to develop products rich in fats, sugar, and salt.

The inability of 'simple' health education, based on numerous government COMA (Committee on Medical Aspects of Food Policy) reports, to decrease the nation's consumption of fats, sugar, and salt, was one of the reasons for the creation of the Food Task Force as part of the Health of the Nation initiative in 1992. The Food Task Force was broadly based and included food manufacturers in order to provide a concerted effort to improve the nation's diet. There have been some successes. Supermarkets and food manufacturers wish now to be seen as 'healthy' and there has been an increase in availability of 'low fat', 'low salt', and 'low sugar' products—at a price.

On a global scale, of considerable concern is the introduction of the worst of western diets into developing countries (e.g. processed foods and drinks, high in fats and sugars at the expense of foods high in complex carbohydrate, fruit, and vegetables) accompanied by western diseases of obesity, diabetes, cardiovascular disease, and caries.

The next section will examine influences on food purchase and consumption in more detail.

## What influences our diet?

The more important influences are given in Table 9.2. It must be recognized that there is much interaction between them: the availability of food will depend on where you live, the distance you are able to travel to purchase the food, how to carry it home, and, in the broader sense, your income available for food purchase. Physical conditions vary enormously between homes as does the knowledge and skills of the cook in the household. Some 60 per cent of women work full or part time, providing less time for food purchases and preparation. Most children eat at school and most working people eat at or near their work at some time of the day. Some of these facilities are excellent, providing good choice of appetizing healthy food, but others are less so.

There has been much debate over whether it is more expensive to eat healthily. Products marketed as low in fat, sugar, and salt are often more expensive than other comparable foods, especially on a per calorie basis (which is important for a hungry family) so that choosing these foods could add to your food bill. Cheaper cuts of meat, and especially many meat products, have a high fat content compared with more expensive cuts of meat. On the other hand potatoes, bread, many vegetables, and some fruits, are relatively cheap. These raw foods may be cheaper than pre-packaged convenience foods but they do require time, skills, and facilities to make them into popular meals. On balance, those working with low income groups have found that eating healthily adds 10 per cent to the food bill. It is important to find ways to reverse this ratio.

There are strong interactions between advertising of food, availability of foods, information given in the media, changing tastes and fashions, and peer pressure. This is seen very strongly in the field of drinks, which are heavily advertised, and much of these advertisements encourage peer pressures—the rise of 'alcopops' in the UK in the late 1990s is an example.

Table 9.2.
Influences on our diet

Availability of food
Living environment
– Home
– School
– Workplace
Price
Changing tastes and fashions
Advertising
Media
– TV
– Newspapers
– Magazines
Peers

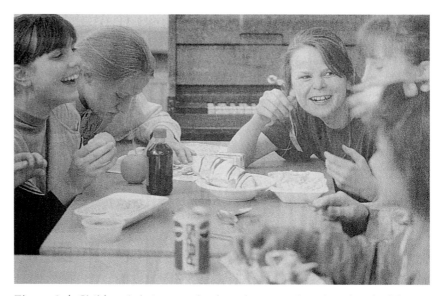

**Figure 9.4** Childrens' choices at school meals—sometimes less than healthy.

It can be appreciated that some of these influences are generated nationally while others exist locally and at an individual level. Each of these will now be discussed in turn.

## National factors

National factors which influence our diet are listed in Table 9.3. Again, there is much interaction between them. For example, government is responsive to pressures from professional organizations, other pressure groups as well as from industry, and would much rather work with these groups than against them. This is one of the key elements of the *Health of the nation* and *Our healthier nation* initiatives.

## Government food policy

For too long in the UK, the two major players influencing what we eat—the Department of Health (DH) and the Ministry of Agriculture, Fisheries and Food (MAFF)—have been at loggerheads. The DH would make pronouncements—eat less fat—but these rarely got translated into action because of the suspicion that MAFF was primarily interested in protecting farming. MAFF is larger and more powerful than the DH and so usually won. Subsidies to farmers for food production have rarely been made on health grounds. Milk producers used to be paid according to the fat content of their milk—the higher the fat the higher the payment. Sugar beet production is still subsidized in the UK and quotas of cane sugar from the Caribbean protected. There have been welcome signs of change over the past few years, beginning with the *Health of the nation* initiative (to which all government departments agreed) and the subsequent formation of the Food Standards Agency

Table 9.3.
National influences on diet

| Government food policy | Department of Health (DH) COMA reports |
| --- | --- |
| | Ministry of Agriculture, Fisheries and Food (MAFF) agriculture policies |
| | The *Health of the nation/Our healthier nation* initiatives |
| | Food Standards Agency (FSA) |
| | School curriculum and school meals |
| | Health education and promotion |
| | Research |
| Legislation and regulation | Food safety (e.g. non-sugar sweeteners) |
| | Food labelling |
| | Food advertising |
| Food industry | Food producers and their generic organizations (e.g. Sugar Bureau, National Alliance of Soft Drink Manufacturers; Biscuit, Cake, Chocolate and Confectionery Alliance; Meat and Livestock Commission) |
| | Supermarkets |
| Professional organizations | British Medical, Dental, and Dietetic Associations |
| | Organizations particularly concerned with children and public health |
| Other pressure groups | National Food Alliance |
| | Consumers Association |
| | Coronary Prevention Group |
| | Caroline Walker Trust |
| | Action and Information on Sugars |
| Media | TV |
| | Press |
| | Magazines |

(FSA). The Agency advises government; it claims that it will put consumers first, have the power to take action, and be independent and open (Box 9.2).

The reports of the Committee on Medical Aspects of Food Policy (COMA) have been much admired for their thoroughness and clarity. COMA is a standing committee of the DH and chaired by the Chief Medical Officer. Those reports relevant to oral health have been discussed in Chapters 7 and 8 and have dictated health education in this country.

It is likely that the work of COMA and health education will come within the remit of the FSA in the future. The Health Education Authority (HEA) has been funded by the DH and has been very supportive of oral health, albeit on a small budget. Their leaflets have been referred to in previous chapters as has been the very influential booklet *The scientific basis of dental health education*, now in its fourth edition.

Box 9.2 **The Food Standards Agency**

'… will have the power to monitor the safety and quality of food. If there is a problem, it will make sure that action is taken to put things right. It will give us the information and advice we need to make sensible choices for ourselves and our families. The Agency will make sure that the arrangements for dealing with food safety in England, Scotland, Wales and Northern Ireland all work to the same standard.'

DH/MAFF (1998)

The major way in which *Our healthier nation* differs from its predecessor *The health of the nation* is in the greater emphasis given to inequalities. Details of how goals are to be achieved have not yet appeared, but it should be remembered that deprived people in society are more likely to eat poorly and have more dental caries and greater tooth loss than more affluent people in society. Health promotion, including diet and water fluoridation, if successfully targeted at the more deprived groups, could improve the oral health of the population substantially.

It is very important that health messages given by health professionals are accurate and consistent. Another important spin-off from the *Health of the nation* was the production in 1994 of the *Core curriculum for nutrition in the education of health professionals*. This document highlights the many deficiencies in the training of doctors, dentists, nurses, and other professions allied to medicine. This report is resulting in increased attention to nutrition and health at the pre-registration level in these professional courses and during continuing professional education.

Government has a central role in determining the school curriculum. Food science and cooking skills have recently been squeezed out of the core curriculum. This is a short-sighted view which could lead to severe loss of cooking skills in the home.

Each of the constituent countries of the UK (England, Scotland, Wales, and Northern Ireland) have published oral health strategies in the past 5 years. Each of these mention diet and the need to reduce sugars consumption.

There has been much emphasis recently on need for health policies to be 'evidence based'. This is quite right, but does mean that the evidence has to be gathered. There has been a very welcome recognition that the National Health Service needs research and development ('R & D') if it is to improve services and improve health. Particularly welcome is the quite large sums of money (over £5 million) made available recently for research in primary dental care in England and Wales. Many of these projects have a dietary aspect and are undertaken by primary dental care staff. Results of these studies should be applicable directly to general dental practice. On a different level, it is very disappointing that less than 3 per cent of the budget of the Medical Research Council is given to nutrition research.

## Legislation and regulation

'Ban smoking' and 'Tax sugar' are easy and well meaning statements to make, but difficult to implement. On the whole, governments do not like legislation—it is cumbersome, time consuming, and smacks of the 'nanny state'. Besides, civil servants would much prefer to maintain the status quo. Government would prefer to give information and allow the consumer to make their own choice. Proponents for health legislation say that this is all very well if the playing fields are level—and often they are far from level. Health legislation has been very successful in some issues, such as seat belts in cars, but near disastrous in others such as water fluoridation. Increasingly, the centre of power for legislation in the area of food and health has moved from London to Brussels.

Food safety was central to the creation of the FSA and will be the most important aspect of its work. Of particular relevance to oral health is the approval of non-sugar sweeteners—these were discussed in Chapter 3 and again in Chapters 7 and 8. There has been a most welcome expansion in the number of non-sugar sweeteners available for use in this and many other countries over the past 10 years. The safety of each of these has been assessed by the Committee on Toxicology (CoT) which advises on their use by the food manufacturer and the public. There are several non-sugar sweeteners whose safety is currently being assessed and, if approved, are very likely to be used as sugar substitutes in foods and drinks. The wider the range of non-sugar sweeteners, the easier it is for food manufacturers to use them since each sweetener has its own properties.

Food labelling is fairly heavily regulated and nutritional labelling is a very important aspect of this. Several professional groups and other pressure groups would say that nutritional labelling regulations are too lax and that the public is not well enough informed on the nutritional content of foods and drinks. A central aspect to this debate is whether labelling should be compulsory or voluntary. At present it is voluntary unless a claim is made. For example, if a claim is made that a product is 'low sugar' then the sugars content has to be given in a standard manner specified by MAFF; likewise, if a claim is made for 'low salt' or 'high fibre'. An example of a nutritional label is given in Fig. 9.5. However, if no claim is made, the manufacturer need not label his product and if he chooses to provide a label, he need not specify sugars content (Fig. 9.6). Such labels are grossly misleading since 69 per cent carbohydrate could mean 69 per cent sugars or 69 per cent starch. The purchaser is pretty well aware that they should decrease sugars consumption but increase starch consumption, yet the label offers no help. Surveys have shown that it is the high sugar products (e.g. confectionery) which are the least well labelled for nutritional content. In this context, the present voluntary arrangement for food labelling is not working.

The confectionery industry spends over £100 million a year on advertising in the UK. This is about 100 times the budget for oral health education in the Health Education Authority. The playing field is not level. Television advertising is expensive and so the food industries have a clear field when it comes to information on television on what to eat. This has caused much concern amongst health professionals and the general public (Box 9.5). Not surprisingly, TV authorities are loath to restrict the amount or content of the advertisements, as this is revenue. The government, for several reasons, is also resistant to action to curb advertising; self-regulation is preferred. The result of self-regulation is weak rules and sometimes disregard for them altogether. Both the Independent Television Commission (ITC) and the Advertising Standards Authority (ASA) have codes of practice (Box 9.6). One of the greatest flaws in the system is they are regulated by *post hoc* complaints. It is only when there is a complaint about an advert that the advertisement is investigated. If the complaint is upheld, the ITC may request withdrawal of the advert but, by then, the damage is largely done. There seems to be considerable scope for further investigation into control of advertising of food and drinks, especially those aimed at children. Some other countries have better controls. Canada does not permit advertising during children's programmes, while in Sweden and Belgium advertisements are banned for 5 minutes before and after children's programmes.

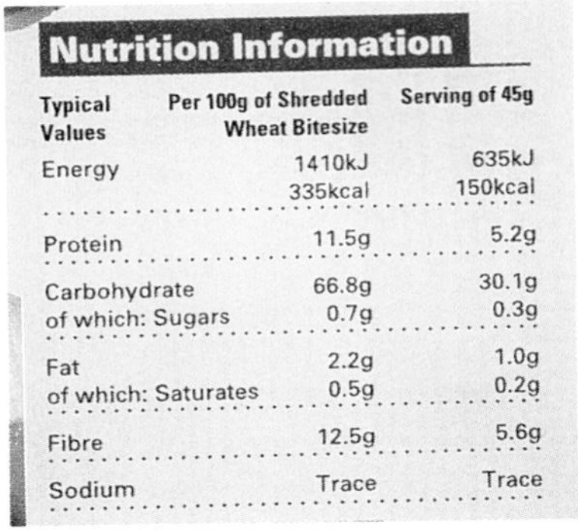

| Nutrition Information | | |
|---|---|---|
| Typical Values | Per 100g of Shredded Wheat Bitesize | Serving of 45g |
| Energy | 1410kJ 335kcal | 635kJ 150kcal |
| Protein | 11.5g | 5.2g |
| Carbohydrate of which: Sugars | 66.8g 0.7g | 30.1g 0.3g |
| Fat of which: Saturates | 2.2g 0.5g | 1.0g 0.2g |
| Fibre | 12.5g | 5.6g |
| Sodium | Trace | Trace |

**Figure 9.5** An example of a nutritional label which gives sugars content.

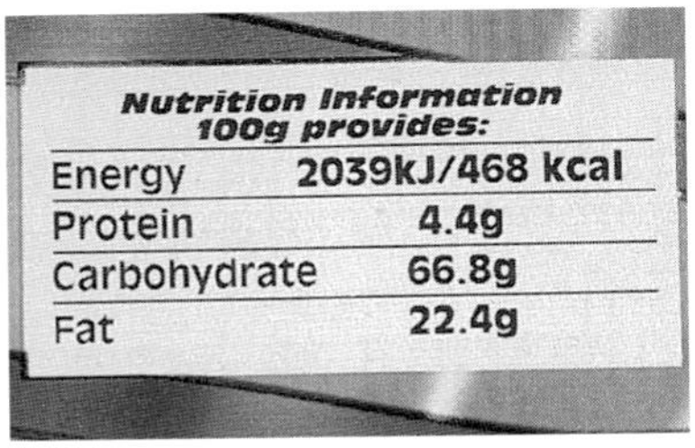

| Nutrition Information 100g provides: | |
|---|---|
| Energy | 2039kJ/468 kcal |
| Protein | 4.4g |
| Carbohydrate | 66.8g |
| Fat | 22.4g |

**Figure 9.6** An example of a label of a confectionery product which does not specify sugars content.

## Box 9.3

A survey of a week's advertisements on UK TV in 1995 found that 60 per cent of advertisements aimed at children were for fatty and sugary foods—while the recommendations are that such foods should make up only 8 per cent of a healthy, balanced diet. There were no advertisements for fruit or vegetables, whereas these should constitute a third of the diet.

National Food Alliance (1996)

## Box 9.4 Advertising and children

- Pre-school children think that the purpose of advertising is to inform, rather than to sell.
- Three quarters of 4 year olds were unable to differentiate between programmes and advertisements.
- Children are more responsive to, and influenced by, advertising than adults.
- Children are a major influence on household food purchases.

National Food Alliance (1996)

## Box 9.6 Independent Television Commission codes of practice

Under 'Health and hygiene':
- Advertisements must not encourage children to eat frequently throughout the day.
- Advertisements must not encourage children to consume food and drink (especially sweet, sticky foods) near bedtime.
- Advertisements for confectionery or snack foods must not suggest that such products may be substituted for balanced meals.

ITC (1991)

## Box 9.5 Public opinion survey conducted by MORI in 1994 for the National Food Alliance

- 'I think there should be tougher restrictions on the advertising of foods and soft drinks to children.'
  64 per cent agreed, 26 per cent disagreed
- 'Current food advertising encourages children to eat a healthy balanced diet.'
  15 per cent agreed, 74 per cent disagreed
- 'I often end up buying advertised foods or drinks which I wouldn't otherwise buy, because my children ask me to.'
  39 per cent agreed, 52 per cent disagreed
- 'Food advertising encourages my children to spend their pocket money on foods I prefer them not to eat.'
  40 per cent agreed, 43 per cent disagreed

A more recent development whose effect has yet to be determined is the sponsorship of TV programmes. This must be seen as a form of advertising.

# Food industry

Industry is an essential part of modern life and the prime reason for our prosperity. The Food Industry has provided attractive, nutritious foods at affordable prices which we are able to buy 365 days of the year. As a slightly tangential point, the toothpaste manufacturers, by their research into the inclusion of fluoride in toothpastes, have done more to improve the dental health of people in the UK than any other single factor. Thus, industry is certainly not all bad. We tend not to like it because it is powerful and its actions appear to be outside our control.

While the activities of the toothpaste industry have definitely been helpful in improving dental health, there are three very powerful industries whose products are detrimental to oral health. These are the sugar and sugar-related industries, for

## Box 9.7 Different views of the role of confectionery in dental disease

One cannot help wondering whether the state of our dental health and especially that of our children is determined much more by Rowntree Mackintosh, Mars and Cadbury Schweppes, than it is by the dental profession.

Chairman, Health Education Council

... normal confectionery consumption does not have a significant influence on the extent of dental decay in the UK.

Cocoa, Chocolate and Confectionery Alliance

their role in promoting consumption of sugar and sugar-containing products—the prime cause of dental caries; and the tobacco and alcohol industries whose products are major risk factors for oral cancer. All three—the sugar and sugar-related industries, the tobacco industry, and the alcohol industry—are very powerful and advertise heavily to maintain or increase sales and market share. Some of the ways in which the sugar-related industries do this are given in Table 9.4. We should not be surprised at this, since this is what their shareholders expect of them. That does not mean that we should accept their action and it is very reasonable that the dental profession seeks to minimize advertising and sales of these products to vulnerable people and educate the public into the damaging effect of tobacco and excessive alcohol and sugar consumption.

The confectionery industry in particular has been active in providing well produced booklets on diet, caries, and oral health. While some of the information in these booklets is good, the information on the role of sugars in oral disease is rather different from that of the Department of Health and the Health Education Authority; in particular, the reliance on tooth-brushing to prevent caries and their contention that all carbohydrates, starch and sugars, are similarly cariogenic.

Although leaders of industry have stated that it is 'not the role of industry to educate the consumer' or 'to seek to improve the health of the general public' there are strong signs that supermarkets are responsive to the public's interest in eating healthily. Leaflets are available and special areas are devoted to organically grown produce or low calorie foods. This is to be encouraged and professions should cooperate with and support these companies to ensure that the advice given is accurate.

## Toothfriendly sweets

Both at a national and at a local level we should encourage industries which are working towards health. There is a definite need for healthier snacks. 'Toothfriendly sweets' go some way towards this. The 'toothfriendly' idea is some 25 years old and began in Switzerland with the development of an intraoral pH telemetric system, which was accepted by the Swiss Health Department as a valid test of non-cariogenicity. Progress became more rapid after 1983, when *Aktion Zahnfreundlich* was established in Switzerland as a partnership between dentists and industry to promote the toothfriendly idea. A logo (Fig. 9.7) was registered and could be displayed on packets of confectionery which had passed the pH test. A small levy was paid on products carrying the logo, which was used for the generic promotion of the toothfriendly idea. By 1991, 20 per cent of confectionery in Switzerland carried the toothfriendly logo, indicating that these products had been shown to be safe, and over 90 per cent of Swiss children knew the meaning of the logo. Since 1983, eight other countries have followed the Swiss lead (Table 9.5) and there are now four test centres to which confectionery manufacturers can apply to have their products tested. Ten years after its introduction, the eye-catching 'Mr happy tooth' may be found on toothfriendly confectionery in more than 20 countries.

The toothfriendly idea is not without its critics: it can be argued that such confectionery is still largely empty calories; polyols are known to cause diarrhoea;

**Table 9.4.** Actions of the sugar-related industries to preserve the sale of sugar in the face of calls for reduced sugar consumption by government and the health professions

Dispute the evidence:
– create uncertainty
– professionals are divided'
– shift the blame (onto starches)
'Soften up' the opposition
'Get at' the decision makers
Heavy advertising

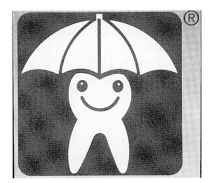

**Figure 9.7** Pictograph of the 'Mr Happy-tooth'. Reproduced with permission of *Toothfriendly International*.

Table 9.5.
Toothfriendly worldwide

| 1983 | Switzerland |
|------|-------------|
| 1986 | Germany |
| 1991 | France |
| 1992 | Belgium |
| 1993 | United Kingdom |
|      | Japan |
| 1994 | Italy |
| 1995 | Korea |
|      | Argentina |

## Box 9.8 Toothfriendly sweets

These sweets have been shown to be non-cariogenic and non-erosive (see Chapter 3). The following products currently carry the logo in the UK:

- Chupa Chups    lollipops
- Detorelle      chews and mints
- Lofthouse      Fisherman's friend mints and pastilles
- Hai Tai        chewing gums
- Ricola         pastilles
- Smint          mints
- Sula           drops
- Velamints      mints

All these products contain polyols such as sorbitol, xylitol, lactitol, maltitol, hydrogenated glucose syrup, and isomalt. If eaten in large amounts, especially by young children, they can cause osmotic diarrhoea so some caution is advisable in their use by young children.

they may encourage a sweet taste; and they are usually more expensive than their sugar-containing counterparts. On the positive side, the test system is now well accepted and very unlikely to pass products which cause caries. Two further reasons are especially important—first, that toothfriendly sweets have substituted for sugar-containing sweets, rather than adding to sales and, second, there would appear to be a positive benefit to dental health. In both Finland and Switzerland, the increased use of non-sugar sweeteners in confectionery appears to have been a factor in the improved dental health of children.

## Box 9.9 British Dental Association food and drinks accreditation

The aim of this scheme is to advise the public of foods and drinks which either positively improve dental health or improve dental health by substitution. This scheme is similar to the 'toothfriendly' initiative but has a broader aim and is limited to the UK. Unlike 'toothfriendly', the BDA approves health claims for products. An example of foods and drinks accredited by the BDA since the launch the scheme in 1998 is

- Ribena Tooth Kind

## Professional organizations

The views of doctors, dentists, and dietitians are important locally in influencing their patient's behaviour and in helping local health promotion activities, but it is their national professional associations which influence national policy. The professions have got themselves much more organized in this respect over the past 10–20 years. Committees such as COMA take opinion from a wide variety of sources and these opinions will be considered carefully when drawing conclusions and making recommendations. The opinions of professional organizations are very important and, indeed, if they are not given when appropriate, it will be taken as a sign of the disinterest of that profession. The end result is that most professional organizations create a bank of policy documents on important topics.

The desirability of reducing sugar consumption is a case in point, with all three professional bodies—the British Medical Association, the British Dental Association, and the British Dietetic Association—all making statements endorsing the Department of Health's view that sugar consumption in the UK should be reduced. The British Medical Association has been in the forefront in the battle to reduce smoking in the UK and the British Dental Association supports this campaign. It is very persuasive if all relevant professions speak with the same voice.

Within the dental profession there is also uniformity, with the most relevant societies—the British Society of Paediatric Dentistry and the British Association for the Study of Community Dentistry—producing policy statements on sugars and dental health.

## Other pressure groups

The effectiveness of these 'pressure groups', such as those listed in Table 9.3, in influencing national policies is unclear. They certainly do good research and their publications are really useful sources of information. It is likely that many decision makers will be persuaded by arguments put forward by these groups. It is tempting to label some of these groups as having a political bias. This is an easy accusation to make but mostly unwarranted since the driving force for the vast majority of these pressure groups is an improvement in health. The National Food Alliance has carried out extensive research on advertising and has produced some very good reports. The Consumer's Association informs the public by publishing the *Which?* magazines. The Coronary Prevention Group has been one of the leading authorities on food labelling, while the Caroline Walker Trust has produced some very good reports (e.g. on school meals) and has done much to bridge the gap between the consumer and the food industry. Much of the easily understood information on the sugar content of foods is produced by Action and Information on Sugars.

One of the most successful campaigns in oral health promotion, organized by pressure groups, is the 'chuck sweets off the checkout' campaign (Fig. 9.8). This campaign was launched in 1992, when over two thirds of supermarket checkouts had confectionery on display, ready to tempt the waiting parent or frustrated child (Fig. 9.9). After the third action day in 1996, the percentage of checkouts with confectionery had fallen to 29 per cent. The top three food retailers in the

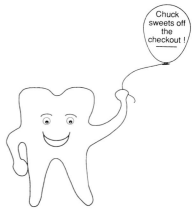

**Figure 9.8** The logo used for the successful 'Chuck the sweets off the checkout' programme in the UK.

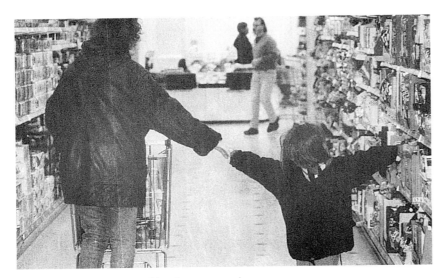

**Figure 9.9** 'Pester-power' in the supermarket.

UK—Tesco, Sainsbury's, and Safeway—all had 100 per cent confectionery-free checkouts, as did the smaller retailer, Waitrose. Sales of confectionery were reported to have fallen by 30 per cent in supermarkets where confectionery had been removed from the checkout.

## The media

The media have been largely responsible in recent years for the increasingly high level of interest in diet and health. Whole magazines are devoted to slimming and many more that specialize in topics related to health regularly feature articles on nutrition. Newspapers, too, frequently feature diet and health, and there are a number of regular television and radio programmes based on food and drink and health. Many of these offer excellent, well balanced accounts, presented in an accessible way, and are undoubtedly highly influential for the good. Others, however, in the drive to present something new, will feature untested nostrums and the theories of unqualified exponents of questionable panaceas.

Acrimonious discussions between 'experts' make for good entertainment and by creative editing and juxtaposition, 'experts' can be ridiculed and the public confused. This can then enable the journalist to appear to be the true defender of the interests of consumers. Minor but topical threats to health can be emphasized out of proportion to their true risk to public health, whilst the main causes of concern are neglected. The media are constantly and effectively used by those with products to defend and sell, but to a lesser extent by health professionals. The health professions need expert help in harnessing the media to promote health effectively.

## Local influences on diet

Local activities to improve diet will depend on national policies to some extent. The role of primary health care is defined nationally, as is the school curriculum. However, there is still much that can be achieved at a local level to encourage better food choice and healthier living. Local conditions, disease prevalence, poverty, attitude of the media and local industry, the enthusiasm of health care workers—all vary enormously across the country, so that it is not surprising that health promotion activities will vary too. The enthusiasm of local health professionals is probably the most important single factor in successful community health promotion.

Activities which influence dietary habits at a local level are listed in Table 9.6. Examples of successful projects can be found under many of these headings, although one of the greatest problems is the lack of adequate evaluation. In these days of evidence-based health care and a greater amount of money being made available for research in primary health care, methods of evaluating health promotion projects are receiving much more attention. One of the most difficult decisions in designing such programmes is to agree on the measurable outcomes. It should be improvement in health and the quality of life, but very often we have to be content with outcomes such as increased awareness, knowledge,

**Table 9.6.**
Local influences on diet

Child and maternity services
Schools
    Curriculum
    School meals
    Tuck shops
Work place
    Industry
    Health service
Primary health care
    General medical practices
    Community health centres
    General dental practices
    Community dietetic services
    Community pharmacists
    Health promotion units
    Health action zones
Media
    TV
    Newspapers
Food retailers
    Supermarkets

increased purchases of more desirable foods, or, better still, change in food consumption. Much work is being done to encourage links between the enthusiastic primary health care worker and experts in design and evaluation (usually in universities) to ensure that findings of projects can contribute to evidence-based health care.

The knowledge and attitudes of midwives and health visitors are important influences on the way a mother will feed her child. Manufacturers of baby drinks and foods are anxious to present free samples to mothers soon after birth—these are often given as 'Bounty Packs'. Local pressures from the dental and dietetic professions can ensure that these are not high-sugar products, as has happened in the past.

While the school curriculum is determined nationally, school meals and tuck shops are very much local issues. Health professionals may well be school governors and can help to determine health policies in schools. The chance to learn cooking skills, the provision of meals in schools, and the choice available in school tuck shops are all issues up for discussion—your expert knowledge is important. There is evidence from Australia and England that banning the sales of sweets in school tuck shops reduces the development of dental caries in children.

Sponsorship is increasing in schools and a worrying factor is the delivery to schools of science portrayed in these packs produced by the sugar industry. The role of sugars in health and disease in these packs is rather different from that given by the Department of Health.

The Health Service is the nation's biggest employer and provides food for patients and staff. Health professions should push for the provision of good attractive foods for their own hospitals and be prepared to be active in promoting health in the workplace.

Seventy five per cent of the UK population visits their general medical practice at least once per year. Incentives encourage health promotion in primary medical care. Continuing education is vital for all health professionals and giving nutritional advice is high on the agenda. Your input into this continuing professional education will be valuable to ensure accurate information on nutrition and oral health. Likewise, the community dental service should be able and willing to advise staff in community health centres and encourage them to promote oral health, working with community dietitians and community pharmacists. Pharmacists are important sources of advice for the public and are likely to welcome your expert advice on dental matters, including dietary aspects of oral diseases.

There is no doubt that the prime responsibility for liaising with the above groups falls on units specifically funded for health promotion. Most communities have health promotion units and some have been very successful at promoting better diets. One of the largest dental health promotion programmes in the UK was undertaken in the North West Region during the early 1990s (Box 9.10). The programme had six components, three of which had important dietary components. A very successful feature of the programme was that it brought different health professionals together to exchange ideas on how health promotion, including healthy eating, could be taken forward in their community. By the

**Box 9.10 Working together to promote dental health**

Some of the components of a health promotion campaign in the North West Region of England, 1988–94.

- Campaign for mothers of young children
- A dental care programme for occasional dental attenders
- Promoting registration of young children
- 'Smile for sugar-free medicines'
- Dental health facilitators
- Working together to put prevention into practice

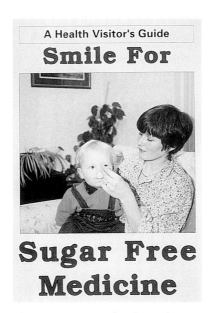

A Health Visitor's Guide

**Smile For**

**Sugar Free Medicine**

**Figure 9.10** Specific advice about sugar-free prescribing in a leaflet for health visitors.

end of the campaign, health visitors were much better informed on dental matters and were much more confident on giving advice on healthy eating to preserve oral health to mothers of young children. To some extent, each of the six projects supported the others and generic posters and leaflets were developed to assist the campaign. Some of the conclusions were that the number of messages to be conveyed in any one project must be very limited—perhaps to one, as in the case of the sugar-free medicines project—and be realistic about the changes you expect to achieve (Fig. 9.10). A full description of this project is given in a 76 page report (see Further Reading). The creation of 'Health Action Zones' by the government, in areas of England with the greatest health problems, should stimulate further inter-professional health promotion programmes.

Community health programmes have been well developed in Scandinavia for a long time. In one survey of the activities of 215 community health centres in Finland, the 323 dental staff devoted 53 per cent of their working time to oral health education. About half of this was for advice targeted at the individual and half for advice given to groups. Virtually all staff included dietary advice, especially the need to avoid frequent sugar consumption. A novel feature of the Finnish campaigns is the encouragement to use xylitol-containing confectionery. One community-based programme involved 6700 children. After a national programme to promote the use of xylitol chewing gum—the 'Smart Habit' campaign—50 per cent of children were using xylitol gum at least once a day; this was maintained 1 month later. Over 95 per cent of the children were aware of the value of xylitol gum in preventing caries.

Programmes to encourage the use of sugar-free confectionery have also been very successful in Switzerland, where 20 per cent of confectionery sold is now toothfriendly. Educational campaigns involve schools and the media and are targeted at both children and parents with considerable success (Box 9.11).

The impact of many of these programmes on dental health is difficult to assess, particularly if the programmes are widespread. A major review of the role of diet in the changing pattern of dental caries in Europe by Professor Marthaler of Zurich University was published in *Caries Research* in 1990. Two paragraphs in the conclusions are given in Box 9.12.

Box 9.11

The Swiss 'Toothfriendly Association' was launched in 1982. Education programmes informed the public of the meaning of the toothfriendly logo. By 1993

- 83 per cent of the Swiss population were aware of the logo
- 98 per cent of children (15–19 years) were aware of the logo
- 20 per cent of those who knew the logo claimed to buy *only* toothfriendly confectionery
- an additional 50 per cent bought toothfriendly products sometimes

Bär (1994).

Box 9.12  **Changing caries prevalence in Europe**

In Southern European countries, sugar consumption has been rising during the last 30 years, and a parallel increase in dental caries prevalence is certain to have occurred. On the other hand, in several highly industrialised countries, consumption of sugar and sweets has remained fairly constant but caries prevalence has been decreasing. This decline of caries prevalence in children is primarily due to the widespread use of fluorides in various forms, most frequently in dentifrices; improved oral hygiene which automatically favours frequent utilization of fluoride-containing products may also have been a factor.

In two cases, however, favourable dietary changes are thought to have occurred: the reduction of caries prevalence in Finnish and Swiss children is not likely to be fully explained exclusively in terms of fluorides and improved oral hygiene. In Finland, the widespread use of xylitol as a sweetener may have been a factor in the improvement of dental health; in Switzerland a lowered cariogenic challenge is suggested by the widespread use of nonacidogenic sweets which already in 1985 constituted 10 per cent of the total of sweets sold.

Source: Marthaler (1990)

# Summary

- Diet has changed and will continue to change. Our role is to encourage change for the better. The UK has good statistics on diet (e.g. the National Food Survey begun in 1940) and dental disease (the 10 yearly national surveys begun in 1968). There have been very welcome improvements in dental health and in some aspects in our diet, but disease levels are still much too high and nutritional intake is too high in fats, sugars, and alcohol and too low in complex carbohydrates, fresh fruit, and vegetables.

- Government has a major role to play in improving diet and oral health. The *Health of the nation*, *Our healthier nation*, and the formation of the Food Standards Agency are hopeful signs of coordinated health promotion at the highest level. Legislation is appropriate to defend public health where voluntary controls have not worked.

- There are several good examples of successful partnerships between health professions and industry: it is much better to find ways to work with industry than against it.

- Professional organizations have a very important role in presenting evidence-based advice to government. It is important that there is un-animity in dietary messages to maintain credibility and avoid confusion.

- Much health promotion can be done at a local level—all members of the dental team have important roles. The most important ingredient in successful local campaigns is the enthusiasm of local professionals. The importance of research in primary dental care is being recognized in the UK. These projects must be properly evaluated if the findings are to be used to promote evidence-based community prevention.

# Further reading

Bentley, E., Brown, C., Fuller, S., Nuttall, J., and Taylor, G. (eds) (1995). *Working together to promote dental health*. North West Region Dental Public Health Resource Centre/FDI World Dental Press, London.

British Society of Paediatric Dentistry (1992). A policy document on sugars and the dental health of children. *Int. J. Paed. Dent.* **2**, 177–80.

British Society of Paediatric Dentistry (1995). A policy document on toothfriendly sweets. *Int. J. Paed. Dent.* **5**, 195–7.

Dibb, S. E. (ed.) (1993). *Children; advertisers' dream, nutrition nightmare?* National Food Alliance, London.

Health Education Authority (1996). *The scientific basis of dental health education. A policy document* (4th edn). HEA, London.

Ministry of Agriculture, Fisheries and Food (1991). *Fifty years of the National Food Survey 1940–1990* (ed. J. M. Slater). HMSO, London.

# 10

# Dietary advice in the dental surgery

# Dietary advice in the dental surgery

## The need for dietary advice

'Dental practitioners should give dietary advice including reduction of non-milk extrinsic sugars consumption as part of their health education to patients, particularly to those who are especially prone to dental caries. To facilitate this, the Panel *recommends* that teaching of nutrition during dental training should be increased, and professional relations between dietitians and dental practitioners be encouraged.'

Paragraph 14.3.9 in 'Conclusions and Recommendations':
Department of Health report,
*Dietary sugars and human disease*,
1989

Since dietary habits are so personal, dietary advice must be personalized if it is to be successful. Such advice is, however, full of pitfalls and needs to be approached in a systematic way. The aim of this chapter is to indicate some of the pitfalls and suggest a systematic yet pragmatic approach in order to enable practitioners to decide whether they are able to offer appropriate advice and when they should ask for help.

## Some influences on dietary habits

We do not eat food simply to satisfy our physiological needs. There is a range of physiological, pathological, psychological, social, economic, and cultural factors which also influence our intake of food (Tables 10.1 and 10.2).

Food and drink, and eating and drinking, have deep symbolic significance; withholding food is universally regarded as a punishment, whilst giving food is a very acceptable reward or gift. Not all foods are regarded in the same light; sweets and chocolates are much more acceptable gifts than apples or mashed potato.

Beliefs about foods are often very strongly held and may reflect religious or moral opinions. Moods can vary dramatically and undoubtedly have strong influences on an individual's food intake. Thus, dietary advice is very often not received or acted upon rationally, and this may give rise to stress since it can cause inner conflict between the desire to be 'healthy' and other perceptions of the role of food.

The cost and availability of food vary greatly, as do priorities with regard to expenditure of family finance. Unemployment is prevalent in some areas and may affect outlook and restrict finance and choice. There are also strong pressures for both young and old people to behave in a similar way to their peers; food habits

### Box 10.1 Role models and peer pressure

Parents have a pivotal role in the nutrition of their children during school years. By precept and example, parents must provide guidance and instil healthy eating habits and attitudes to foods and eating. Home diets should encourage regular meal eating providing variety, balance, and moderation in nutrient intakes. Getting up in good time to prepare and eat breakfast is important.

Away from home, peer pressure has a considerable influence on eating habits in older children. Sensible parents will accept this reality, encouraging sensible and enjoyable eating at home and giving advice and help in obtaining better food choice in schools and elsewhere.

are one way of reinforcing group identity. Ethnic minority groups may preserve their identity in part by adhering to 'traditional' eating habits. To suggest changes to such habits, therefore, may be to invite criticism.

Table 10.1.
## Some common physiological and pathological conditions which may affect nutritional requirements or dietary habits

| Physiology | Pathology |
| --- | --- |
| Pregnancy | Obesity |
| Lactation | Diabetes mellitus |
| Growth | Hypertension |
| Hard physical exercise | Coronary heart disease |
|   Work | Mental illness |
|   Sport | Anaemia |
| Stress | Poor growth or weight loss |
| Sedentary lifestyle | Carcinomas |
|   Choice | |
|   Imposed | |
| Old age | |

Table 10.2.
## Some circumstances which may affect dietary habits

Cultural factors: ethnicity, religion, vegetarianism
Unemployment
Occupation (e.g. in food industry)
Working unsocial hours (e.g. shift work or long hours)
Excessive travelling to work or school
Unsatisfactory accommodation (e.g. bedsit, overcrowding)
Poor food storage facilities, no refrigerator
Poor cooking facilities (e.g. shared)
Inability to cook
Remoteness from shops (e.g. lack of transport, personal or public; reliance on
   mobile shops)
Poor choice and quality of foods in available shops
Poor choice or dependence on workplace or school for meals
Financial problems
Stress, e.g. divorce, illness
Lack of desire to cook/eat (e.g. elderly, single people)

# Case report

Harry is an only child, aged 7 years, whose mother is a Health Visitor. She is determined that Harry does not eat any 'rubbish' and made all his meals when he was a baby, avoiding the use of any colourants in foods. Unfortunately Harry eats sporadically, has frequent illnesses, and, all in all, is not the healthiest of specimens. His dental downfall is that he was breastfed until nearly three years of age. The pattern of caries is classical—nursing caries syndrome—with incisors and first primary molars the first affected. Harry has had one general anaesthetic to have three of these first primary molars removed—not a good introduction to dentistry. Weaning him from his dependence on his mother was not easy—sometimes it needs something dramatic, like his mother going away for a few days or an extended few days in hospital, as a catalyst for change. The downside of forcing a child into what is essentially an adult way of eating is that the child becomes furtive about 'forbidden' foods, and clears the decks of sweet foods at friends' parties or hoards sweets and biscuits when he can get hold of them, to eat secretly. Rationing treats is a more sensible approach and giving the child some choice in the matter may help establish sensible eating; putting all their treat foods into a box which they can eat from once or twice a week—perhaps after lunch on a Saturday and maybe one evening after tea during the week. Party bags, other presents, and pocket money purchases then can go into the 'sweetie box'.

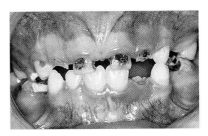

**Figure 10.1** The effects of prolonged breastfeeding, especially if it is after 12 months of age, on demand, and overnight.

## Box 10.2 'Muesli belt malnutrition'

In the UK during the 1980s, a few well meaning parents took the 'healthy eating' message of 'decrease fat and increase fibre' too far, applying this severely to their very young children. Young children need food for growth and some fat in the diet is essential. Semi-skimmed milk should not be given to children under 2 years of age and skimmed milk not before the age of 5 years. High-fibre diets are not well tolerated by young children, inhibiting absorption of some nutrients and possibly resulting in malnutrition.

In recent years, the nature of the family has undergone radical changes. Family units have become smaller, couples have fewer children; there are more one-parent families; ties with relatives seem to be weaker and more mothers work outside the home, and some students are now seriously poor. Finally, there have also been considerable changes in food technology—for example the development of the microwave oven and many forms of 'convenience' foods. These factors all contribute to current food habits, with convenience being a priority apparently often ahead of health. Recognized meal patterns are giving way to 'grazing'.

Dental caries in developed countries is most prevalent in the least affluent communities where the widest variety of the most serious problems listed in Table 10.2 are to be found. In short, eating habits in general and dental conditions in particular may be the least of the family's concerns.

## Box 10.3 Saturday Sweets Day

Sweets are much more than just another food: sweet foods have been valued as gifts for centuries in nearly every culture. In some areas of the UK, sweets are 'kets'—a form of currency. Traditionally, they have all too often been used as a reward. Therefore to ban sweets completely is unrealistic. Since frequency of consumption of sugars is so important in caries aetiology, Scandinavian preventive dentists devised the idea of Saturday Sweets Day. This allows sweets to be accumulated during the week and eaten at one time—after lunch on a Saturday may be a convenient time. This has the advantage of dramatically reducing frequency of sugar exposure without inducing a feeling of deprivation and resentment.

# Dietary advice

Giving dietary advice successfully, therefore, depends on far more than providing knowledge; it requires sensitive understanding of the role of food in society and its significance for the individual patient. Dietary advice consists of several distinct elements which are detailed below: it cannot be considered a one-off event—the provision of simple factual information. Changing eating habits is one of the most difficult changes in behaviour to achieve because of the all-pervasive nature of food. It may involve challenging the beliefs of the entire 'family' and certainly modifying several aspects of lifestyle. Ideally, changes in food-related behaviour should be paralleled by changes in other aspects of health-related behaviour in order to produce a healthier person in all respects. Although this may be impractical for the average busy general practitioner to initiate, it should always be borne in mind that food habits are only one factor in health promotion.

The patient's receptivity to advice varies with, amongst other things, their mood and sense of urgency; giving advice during a time of crisis—for example after a dental extraction—may result in hearty agreement and promises, which are not realistic. The substance of the advice is unlikely to be absorbed or remembered accurately.

The ability to implement even simple advice such as 'eat more fresh fruit' may depend upon factors completely outside the control of the individuals concerned. Advice which cannot be followed is not just unproductive but could be counterproductive as it may lead to a feeling of failure with lowered self-esteem, and hence to the individual deciding to quit the 'system'. Advice has to be personal, practical, and positive.

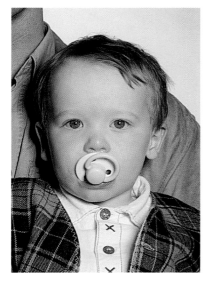

**Figure** 10.2 The dummy in place—with the flange *inside* the lower lip.

## Case report

Shaun is a pre-school child who is reluctant to give up his dummy. He has it when he goes to bed and, on occasions, when he is tired. Although he does not have anything on the dummy now, he used to have it dipped in jam. The consequences are there to be seen. He has rampant caries affecting the majority of his erupted teeth and gross caries of all his incisors. In addition, there is an anterior open bite. The unusual feature about the use of the dummy is that Shaun uses it with the flange inside his lower lip. Whilst not producing any damage at the moment, this is potentially harmful to the soft tissues. Management consists of ensuring first of all that Shaun is pain-free and then dealing with his caries. Whilst the use of the dummy at this stage is not to be condoned, provided it is not dipped in anything, it can be continued. The anterior open bite will resolve once the habit ceases. The parents need to be counselled about the way the dummy is used as well. If the habit were to persist, then the parents could arrange to 'lose' the dummy, preferably late at night when there is no prospect of buying a replacement. A few disturbed nights can be expected, but that should see the issue resolved. Some people would take the view that stopping a habit such as this prematurely predisposes to the child adopting other, perhaps less desirable habits, such as bed-wetting, in a previously continent child. There is, however, no evidence to support this.

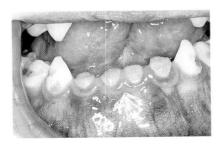

**Figure 10.3** The effects on the dentition of the child in Fig. 10.2 of a dummy that has been coated with sweet foods.

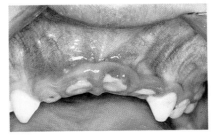

**Figure 10.4** The anterior open bite as well as rampant caries in the child in Fig. 10.2.

Box 10.4 **Use of a dummy**

Suckling is natural in infants and is necessary for survival. Some non-nutritive suckling can be expected and is likely to involve the thumb or a dummy. Long-term studies have not associated the use of a dummy with any adverse oral effects— as long is it is clean, well made, and not dipped in food. Dipping dummies into honey or jam has obvious adverse dental effects. Poorly made dummies can strip gingivae and lacerate the oral mucosa.

# Towards changing behaviour

The general dental practitioner needs to persuade his or her patients to want to change their behaviour. The ability to persuade a patient to change his or her behaviour depends on the effectiveness of communication with that patient. Briefly, communication as a means of persuasion is regarded as comprising 'source factors', 'message factors', and 'audience factors'. These may then result in the recipient changing his or her opinions, perceptions, and/or action.

## Source factors

Source factors are, in this case, those characteristics of the practitioner such as his or her expertise, trustworthiness, likeability, status, race, and religion. The practitioner should be knowledgeable and project trustworthiness (through a confident approach and not making exaggerated claims) and 'likeability' by being sympathetic and patient.

## Message factors

The message factors include how the information is put, the order in which arguments are given and whether both sides of the argument are presented, the types of appeal, and whether the conclusions are explicit or implicit. Any suggestion of 'nagging' should be avoided. The use of fear (e.g. of loss of teeth) is popular; while it may work in the short term, its long-term effectiveness is doubtful. Status can be developed and signalled via the surroundings and the maintenance of high standards of professional conduct. The message, consisting of arguments and evidence, should be rehearsed beforehand and the importance of a consistent approach is stressed.

## Audience factors

Audience factors, that is the patient, include his or her persuasability, initial position, intelligence, self-esteem, and personality factors. The audience factors will have to be assessed but, apart from being aware of the need to maintain self-esteem, are not subject to change although the presentation of the message may vary accordingly. It may be expected that a patient's attention will be high in a surgery setting but comprehension may well be poor despite individual tuition. Only a limited amount of information should be provided at any one time and comprehension should be checked by questioning and re-checked at subsequent visits. Whether or not the patient accepts the messages offered may well not be clear and this may be the major stumbling block preventing change. The extent of change achieved must be monitored at subsequent visits. Most people like to think of themselves as able to make up their own minds and, if there is a feeling that someone is trying to take that away, 'reactance' will occur and will become a barrier to further progress.

Trying to change behaviour is complex but it is certainly much more than just giving advice. It requires an accurate appraisal of the needs, circumstances, and the ability of the patient to change. Above all it requires that the patient wishes to change.

## Case report

Andrea, aged 35 years, has just moved to the area and has attended because of pain from her teeth (Figs 10.5, 10.6). This is her fifth move in 8 years and settling herself and her family as well as a new job have meant that she has adopted a chaotic lifestyle. Andrea is heavily reliant on child-minders to take care of the children for limited periods while she works, leaving little time for cooking and shopping at the end of each day. The family are heavily reliant on convenience foods—ready prepared meals—with little in the way of fresh fruit and vegetables. Andrea tends to snack a lot—when she gets to work, the canteen has tempting snacks to replace the missed breakfast and more snacks, usually biscuits, while the meal is being prepared in the evening because by then she is really hungry. Because her work involves moving around the area she works from, lunch may only be a sandwich or even confectionery—it is easier to eat!

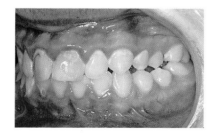

**Figure 10.5** White spot lesions and recurrent caries in a patient who has neglected her mouth and snacked frequently.

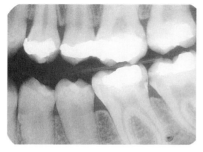

**Figure 10.6** The bitewing radiograph for the left side of the patient in Fig. 10.5 showing the recurrent caries—a high risk patient.

Your role is to persuade Andrea to adopt a healthier way of living, as well as eating. She needs to put herself first and see that, although the way she lives works in the short term, in the long term it is not good for the family's general and dental health. As with many patients, it is not only the family member in the chair that your advice affects, but others too.

## Box 10.5 **Stress, eating, and drinking**

Stress can affect diet adversely—meals are missed or hurried and meal planning may become less important. Snacking or 'eating on the hoof' may become more prevalent and confectionery may be resorted to 'to provide energy for the brain'. Alcohol consumption may also increase with stress—to calm nerves and induce sleep. Comfort bingeing may occur, so may gastrointestinal problems which can result in changed diet and oral medication. These are very difficult cases to deal with, although sugar-free confectionery will help to lessen the threat of rampant caries for continuous sweet-eaters.

Any patient with a heavily restored dentition and evidence of a number of new lesions may need to have their whole lifestyle investigated. Patients often report that writing out a 3 day dietary record is quite salutary—they never realized what they were eating!

Alongside managing dietary change goes aggressive prevention with fluorides to halt the caries progression, at least until the patient is in a lower risk category.

# Dietary advice

## General advice

Advice can be considered to be on two levels. First, some advice should be given to all patients as part of your general preventive care. Leaflets are a great help here—especially those produced by the Health Education Authority (in England and Wales), the Health Education Board for Scotland, and the Health Promotion Agency for Northern Ireland. Seek out your local Health Education Office and discuss the choice of leaflets with them. Some commercially sponsored leaflets are also excellent but do check these carefully to ensure that the messages are sound.

Equally important to giving advice is giving the patient the opportunity to ask questions. One of the important side-effects of media attention to eating is their love of creating controversies (which can be seen in many television programmes); you can do much to reassure your patients as to the correct advice. If you are unsure of some aspects, ask the British Dental Association for advice (Tel. 0171-935-0875).

## Advice to patients at high risk of developing oral disease

Patients who present with high caries experience or extensive dental erosion must be considered for detailed dietary advice. This will involve you and the patient in considerable time. However, if dietary changes are not made, disease will progress, your patient will question your ability to provide oral care, and you could risk legal action for negligence (Fig. 1.1). If they achieve dietary change, the patient's perception of you will be enhanced and you will have helped to improve their oral and general health—possibly of their family also.

## Box 10.6 **Pregnancy**

Pregnancy can be a particularly receptive time for advice on health, both for the mother and the baby. Messages given and targets set now are more likely to be met and can represent a major change in behaviour. Dietary advice for the mother-to-be should be especially guarded and individuals should be referred to the dietician if there is any evidence at all of irregular dietary habits or nutritional problems. Cravings for sweet foods are relatively commonplace during pregnancy—such cravings should pass and are unlikely to do much harm. The importance of oral hygiene should be stressed, to prevent the onset or exacerbation of pregnancy gingivitis, along with the importance of not missing meals and of eating a varied diet that is low in fat, sugar, salt, and alcohol and high in starch, fresh fruit, and vegetables. Do stress that changes made now should be maintained, to bring lifelong benefit to the patient and her family.

## Case report

Judith attended her dentist complaining of sensitivity of her teeth. She is 22 years old and had been a regular attender for many years but latterly had lapsed and was attending after a number of years without any dental attention. When sitting in the dental chair, although well hidden by a bulky sweater and loose-fitting trousers, she appeared thin. On clinical examination her oral hygiene was scrupulous and there was no evidence of dental caries. What was evident was the marked recession on the buccal surfaces of her teeth which accounted for the symptoms of sensitivity (Figs 10.7 to 10.9). Questioning about oral hygiene habits indicated that a too vigorous horizontal scrub technique was being used. Dietary investigations into the possibility of erosion proved fruitless, with an apparently normal diet as detailed on the dietary record completed by the patient. In fact, Judith had anorexia nervosa.

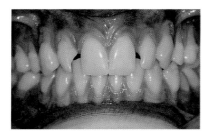

**Figure** 10.7 The marked recession evident on the buccal and labial surfaces of the permanent teeth in the patient (Case report—Judith) with scrupulous oral hygiene but faulty technique. Obsessive behaviour like this is characteristic of patients with eating disorders.

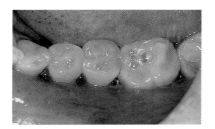

**Figure** 10.8 Eroded, 'cupped' areas affecting the occlusal surfaces of the premolar and molar teeth in this patient with anorexia nervosa.

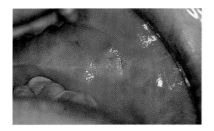

**Figure** 10.9 Keratotic lesions in the buccal mucosa as a consequence of sharp buccal margins from adjacent eroded teeth. These are sometimes seen on the lateral borders of the tongue.

In cases like this the dentist cannot and should not try and solve the problem on his or her own. Such patients need skilled psychiatric care and support from the dental team. The expertise of a dietitian may also be needed. Your role is to make sure that the environment is non-threatening to the patient—or she will not return. Most patients refuse to acknowledge that they have an eating problem and certainly will not be prepared to divulge this to a dentist. Dealing with the signs and symptoms of the disease is the next priority. Modification of brushing habits and generalized, tentative advice about eating patterns are probably all that you can hope to achieve. Restoration of the abrasion/erosion cavities (Figs 10.7, 10.8) may well be indicated because of sensitivity and/or the use of desensitizing toothpastes and a daily fluoride mouthwash. Binge vomiting may be a feature of the condition and, to an extent, the distribution of the tooth surface loss will give you a clue about this—palatal surfaces of upper molar teeth and the occlusal and buccal surfaces of lower molar and premolar teeth may show signs of erosive wear. An empathetic attitude on behalf of the dental team will keep the patient in attendance and ensure that you have the opportunity to minimize the potential for dental harm.

## Stages of dietary advice

A successful system for giving dietary advice involves the completion by the patient of a dietary diary. Three stages are necessary, which can coincide with appointments for other dental care:

1. Obtain a good medical and social history. Give out the dietary record form.

### Box 10.7 **Body weight issues**

Years ago it was popular to distinguish between the poor, who were expected to be those who suffered solely from problems of dietary inadequacy, and more affluent groups whose problems were assumed to consist primarily of disorders associated with dietary excess. Such distinctions are no longer valid in developed countries. In certain subgroups of adolescents, such as teenage girls, emaciation due to anorexia nervosa is more common among the more affluent and obesity is more common among the poor.

Adolescents themselves, especially girls, often have an extremely unrealistic view of what they look like and how they can change their body shapes by gaining or losing weight. Often there is no health reason for doing so. Excessively lean teenagers who may need special help include teenagers suffering from anorexia nervosa, a form of self-induced starvation due to psychiatric causes. Obese adolescents need help to reduce their fatness. Physical activity is to be encouraged in all adolescents. The goal of dietary treatment is not weight loss but fat loss and the growth of lean tissue. In most cases a programme that includes social and psychological support of the obese adolescent, modest calorie reductions, and a vigorous physical activity programme that expends energy, favours the development of muscles and bones, and includes a social component, is more likely to be successful. Anorexic or bulimic patients need professional psychiatric help. A dentist can do much to help the patient appreciate that this is desirable and to assist referral.

2. Receive back the completed diet record.

3. Give advice based on analysis of the diet record. Encouragement and support at subsequent appointments is essential.

## General history including medical and social history

A history of the rapidity of the caries or erosion attack will help you to determine whether the adverse dietary factors are current or previous, and their severity. An accurate record of the current disease level is important in order to judge progression of the disease—written records are essential; radiographs, photographs, and models can be very useful. The opinion of the patient (and parent) about their teeth is important in judging motivation and expected cooperation. If you perceive that the level of cooperation is likely to be very low, you may consider that detailed dietary analysis and advice is impractical—but you must explain and record this outcome.

### Medical history

A list of common conditions requiring special consideration is given in Table 10.1. Any advice offered must not conflict with advice necessary to treat or prevent recurrence of any other nutritionally related problems. An anaemic patient should not be discouraged from eating meat, whilst a patient losing weight pathologically may need to eat more fatty and sugary foods. It should always be established whether the patient has previously received advice from any other source—for example dietitians, doctors, or nurses, and, if so, what it was. Caution is required if there is any doubt and the patient's medical practitioner's opinion sought.

### Socioeconomic history

It is important to try to establish the degree of choice possible for the family and to avoid offering impractical or unwelcome advice. Some relevant socioeconomic circumstances are summarized in Table 10.2. Factors which are related to food intake, but which are not readily subject to change must be identified, in order to indicate the scope for change. Particular care must be taken to identify ethical, cultural, and religious reasons for dietary habits. Financial constraints and access to shops providing a variety of good quality foods must also be assessed. The number in the family, their ages, its structure, whether the adults are working, the cooking and food storage facilities available, and who looks after the children, should all be noted. Any problems in these areas are likely to take precedence over eating habits and advice should be tailored accordingly.

---

## Box 10.8 **Illness**

Illness can affect food habits in a variety of ways. Intake may fall, the choice of foods may change or be imposed, as may frequency of intake. During illness, frequent intakes of confectionery and soft drinks are often encouraged by relatives and friends anxious to show their concern and affection. Unfortunately, illness is also likely to coincide with a decline in oral hygiene, especially when hospitalized. Gifts other than confectionery can be substituted. Sugar-free medicines, prescribed or over-the-counter, should be used whenever possible.

Diet therapy may affect the texture of the diet, the amounts of specific nutrients consumed, and pattern of consumption. There are some disorders which are specifically treated with diets and which are required to have a high content of sugars in order to maintain energy intake (see also Chapters 7 and 8).

---

## Case report

Danielle is 2.5 years old. At a screening in her nursery, the dental officer noted caries of her front teeth and suggested that her mother make an appointment for dental care. Danielle has had no pain from these teeth. The family lives in a non-fluoridated area. Danielle is a 'picky' eater according to her mother. Danielle is happy enough to sit in the chair. Clinical examination reveals a typical pattern of decay referred to as 'nursing caries', with maxillary incisors and first primary molars (Fig. 10.10), usually uppers, affected. While these teeth are symptomless, they can be left whilst more fundamental issues are sorted out. Danielle's mother is asked to complete a 3 day dietary record for her daughter and topical fluoride varnish is applied to the affected teeth. No more than this should be attempted at this visit. On return, Danielle's diet leaves a lot to be desired and what she eats at nursery is a mystery. This needs to be verified. One good, positive item to tell her mother is that there should be no food or drinks close to bedtime. After that there is less to be positive about. The diet lacks sufficient of the basic nutrients and there is plenty of cariogenic challenge. Danielle's mother needs help to get her daughter eating well. For example, breakfast of cereal and/or toast with butter or margarine would be desirable. Children as young as this should not be on low-fat diets until they are school-age. Substituting the sweetened tea with milk would also be a step in the right direction but Danielle may balk at this. An alternative would be to have artificial sweeteners in her tea but this is undesirable on two counts: giving non-sugar sweeteners to toddlers is not desirable and it just keeps Danielle liking a sweet taste rather than re-educating her palate, albeit slowly. Those obvious elements apart, there are more fundamental issues on the diet to be sorted out and this is the sort of case where you would need to get a dietitian's help. Your local hospital will have a dietetics department but you should first see if Danielle's general medical practice provides a dietetic service. This is the time to suggest fluoride supplements. Danielle's mother has returned despite the indicators to the contrary at the previous visit—no history of regular attendance, first visit of pre-school child with extensive caries, poor diet, no fluoride supplements to date. At this age, Danielle could be given a 0.5 mg fluoride tablet for daily use (Box 7.10, page 118). Instructions would be to allow the tablet to dissolve slowly and, if possible, let it dissolve on different sides of the mouth each successive day. If they miss a day, do not double up the dosage next day. At the same time, Danielle should be having her teeth brushed for her, certainly before she goes to bed, and in the morning after breakfast if possible too. She should be using a fluoride toothpaste and, at this stage, provided there is good compliance with the supplement use, a children's variety, maximum 500 ppm fluoride (equivalent to approximately 0.4 per cent sodium monofluorophosphate or 0.1 per cent sodium fluoride), as a pea-sized amount. If compliance proves to be poor with the supplements, then move on to using an adult version toothpaste to give better protection to the dentition. Inevitably, at this age, there will be some systemic absorption until Danielle is old enough to rinse and spit out.

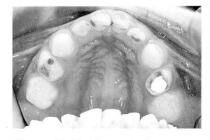

**Figure 10.10** The typical distribution of caries in the primary dentition in a child who has 'nursing caries syndrome', with maxillary incisors and both maxillary and mandibular first primary molars affected initially.

## Determination of usual eating habits

If the evaluation of the information so far indicates that further discussions about diet are likely to be helpful, then an assessment of the patient's eating habits should be made if at all possible. This will enable advice to be personalized and hence to be more relevant to the individual and so more likely to be acted upon.

There are three methods for recording an individual's intake. First, the individual may be asked to recall what they have eaten over a period of time, usually the previous 24 h. Second, the individual may be asked to recount their usual dietary habits for a typical week. Finally, the individual may be asked to keep a record of everything they actually eat for a given period; perhaps three consecutive days or a week.

The '24 h recall' is of little value since the previous day may be very atypical, memory is very unreliable, and the temptation to improve on one's intake is irresistible. The 'usual consumption method' (or diet history) is of more use

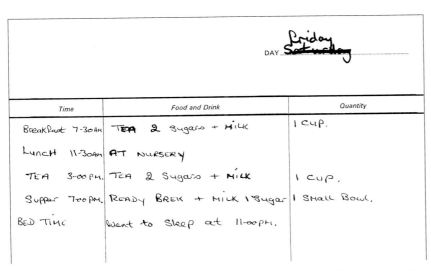

Figure 10.11 A page from the 3 day dietary record for the child in Fig. 10.10.

since, by definition, it is 'typical' but is still prone to memory lapses and to 'talking a better diet'. In addition, dietary interviews are often best carried out by someone experienced in dietetics, and they can be time consuming.

The most appropriate method is to ask the patient to keep a record of intake—although the record may still be a reflection of what the patient thinks you want to hear, it should eradicate lapses of memory and the process itself is informative. Many patients who have kept records comment that they did not appreciate just what or how much they were eating. The method is still prone to be atypical but this can be discussed with each patient. Patients who fabricate their accounts of what they eat may or may not be aware of what they have done. It is unwise to challenge them directly about inconsistencies and the account should be accepted at face value since a 'successful' challenge may lead to alienation.

In deprived areas, where illiteracy is high and motivation low, diet recall could be more appropriate: at the least, it will provide an opportunity to talk to the patient sympathetically and hence to begin to form a productive working relationship.

## Giving out the dietary record sheet

This is the most important stage and involves two components. First, you have to motivate the patient to complete the dietary record. They need to appreciate why they should do it and how it will help you to help them. They have the problem but you have the expert knowledge to help them. Explain to the patient (and parent) that completing a dietary record will involve them in much work for 3 days—don't underestimate this. Second, you should ensure that they understand how to complete the record form (shown in Figs 10.12 and 10.13). Go through each line of the first page ensuring that they understand what is required. Point out the three pages for each of the three days to be recorded, and the requirement to record the time of consumption, what was eaten, and how

| DIET RECORD | RECORD NUMBER |
| --- | --- |
| STAFF: ..................................................... | SURNAME |
| | FIRST NAMES |
| DATED: ..................................................... | DATE OF BIRTH |

Write down in detail all foods and drinks taken for THREE consecutive days, including *everything taken between meals*. This will help us to estimate the properties of the present diet.

Either record the days Thursday, Friday and Saturday **or** Sunday, Monday and Tuesday.

It is important that the times of meals and snacks be noted and whether any of these are eaten away from home (e.g. at school).

Please also put down the time of going to bed

**Suggested Ways of Measuring some of the Foods Used**

| | |
| --- | --- |
| MILK, AND OTHER DRINKS | in tablespoons, cups or tumblers |
| BREAKFAST CEREALS | in tablespoons or cups |
| BREAD | in slices (large or small loaf, brown or white bread) |
| POTATOES | in tablespoons, or compare with an egg |
| SUGAR | tea, dessert or tablespoons |
| MILK PUDDINGS OR CUSTARD | in tablespoons |
| BISCUITS | number and type |
| JAM ETC. | in teaspoons |
| SWEETS, CHOCOLATE, ICE CREAM | cost, size or number |
| MEDICINES | teaspoons |
| 'POP' OR CORDIALS | glasses or cups |

**Figure 10.12** The front page of the 3 day dietary record detailing how the information should be recorded.

much (in household measures). The time of bed should be entered for each of the 3 days. Indicate the importance of recording everything, even a glass of water and any medications taken, either prescribed or over-the-counter medicines. Dietary habits differ between weekdays and weekend days and the scheme allows for the recording of one weekend day and two weekdays.

It is important not to get drawn into giving advice at this stage. Deflect questions by saying that it is better to look at the whole diet and this is what the dietary record form is for. Especially, do not criticize eating habits at this stage as it will create guilt and may well affect the completion of the record.

| Time | Food and Drink | Quantity |
|------|----------------|----------|
|      |                |          |
|      |                |          |
|      |                |          |
|      |                |          |
|      |                |          |
|      |                |          |
|      |                |          |
|      |                |          |
|      |                |          |
|      |                |          |

DAY.................................................

**Figure 10.13** A page from the 3 day dietary record with columns clearly laid out indicating where to record the *time* of the intake, a description of the *type* of food or drink consumed, and lastly, the *amount*. Time of going to bed should also be recorded.

## Receiving the form back

This is the shortest stage. First, it is essential to praise the patient and appreciate the effort they have made. Second, go through the diet record carefully with the patient to ensure that it is adequately filled in. For example, have bedtimes been entered, did a 'cup of tea' have milk and sugar added? What did 'a sandwich' contain? If 'orange juice' is recorded, is this fresh orange juice or diluted fruit squash and, if the latter, is it a low-sugar, sugar-free or sweetened squash? If there are long gaps with no intake recorded, gently question what happened at these times. You can appreciate the advantages of the three stages—giving out the dietary sheet, receiving the dietary sheet back, and giving advice—being fairly close. A week between each of the three stages is about optimum.

## Diet analysis

This is not done in the patient's presence but at some other time. It will take about 15 minutes and you will need another form (Fig. 10.14). This form is in two halves. The top half is concerned with eating habits and sugar control, while the lower half is concerned with the general properties of the diet. Your advice will combine these two aspects. You will see that the top half has four questions.

• **How many intakes per day and how many of these were meals?** Defining an intake precisely is impossible, but the question is asked to help categorize people into meal-eaters or grazers. Generally, meals are more desirable and contain better quality foods. The following descriptions may be useful:

Meal: an intake of food which makes a substantial contribution to the individual's daily intake; which consists of several food groups; which is likely to consist of more than one course and should include a savoury course. The items of which the meal consists are likely to require some preparation, cutlery to consume, and its consumption is likely to be a social activity.

Snack: an intake of food or drink which, by itself, makes a minor contribution to overall intake of useful nutrients (although a day's snacks added together may account for most, if not all, of the intake); requires very little or no preparation and no cutlery to consume; and the consumption of which is a minor activity, often taking place whilst engaged in other activities.

• **How many of these contain sugar?** You should look at this from a public health viewpoint, not a purely biochemical viewpoint. Even bread contains sugars but, overall, bread is not a threat to teeth and is a valuable food. Look for foods which clearly contain a significant proportion of non-milk extrinsic sugars—confectionery, sugar-containing soft drinks, sugar in tea and coffee, biscuits and cakes, and so on. By combining this information with that obtained on the first two lines of this top table you can see whether the patient is a meal-eater or a snacker and whether or not these intakes usually contain non-milk extrinsic sugars or acid drinks or foods.

• **Was a sugar-containing food eaten within 1 h of bed?** Salivary flow virtually ceases during sleep. As explained in Chapter 3, saliva is very important in clearing sugars from the mouth and especially at raising the pH in dental plaque. Plaque pH curves following sugar eating usually last about 30–60 minutes and if a patient goes to sleep within this period, the pH of the plaque is likely to stay low for many hours. This may be especially harmful. While it is true that scrupulous teeth cleaning can remove plaque, it is best to ignore the effect of tooth-brushing (although of course encourage tooth-brushing) as we know that most patients are incapable of removing all plaque.

By completing the analysis for each day and averaging the values over 3 days, you will have a good idea of the pattern of eating of the patient and how this may effect their teeth.

| DIET ANALYSIS | | | | | | RECORD NUMBER |
|---|---|---|---|---|---|---|

**DIET ANALYSIS**

**ANALYSIS OF DIET RECORD**

STAFF: ......................................

DATED: ......................................

RECORD NUMBER

SURNAME

FIRST NAMES

DATE OF BIRTH

AGE:                                                    RECOMMENDATIONS

| EATING HABITS AND NME SUGARS CONTROL | DAY 1 | DAY 2 | DAY 3 | AVERAGE | RECOMMENDED MAXIMUM |
|---|---|---|---|---|---|
| Number of times food is taken each day | | | | | Not more than 6 |
| Number of snack intakes | | | | | up to 3 but none containing NME sugars |
| Number of intakes containing NME sugar | | | | | Not more than 3 |
| NME sugar within 1 hour of bedtime | | | | | None |

| DIET IN GENERAL | SERVINGS PER DAY | | | AVERAGE | SUGGESTED FOODS |
|---|---|---|---|---|---|
| | DAY 1 | DAY 2 | DAY 3 | SUGGESTED | |
| STARCHY FOODS | | | | | Bread, rice, pasta, maize, breakfast cereal, potatoes, noodles |
| | | | | 5 or more | |
| FRUIT | | | | | Fresh, frozen, canned. Oranges, apples, pears, berries (natural juices). *Natural fruit juices and canned fruit contain NMES. |
| | | | | 3 or more* | |
| VEGETABLES | | | | | All fresh, frozen and canned. |
| | | | | 3 or more* | |
| POULTRY/MEAT/FISH/ EGGS, nuts, beans, pulses | | | | | Preferably lean; have fish twice a week if possible |
| | | | | 2-3 | |
| MILK/CHEESE | | | | | Choose low-fat varieties, preferably skimmed. Can be made up (sauces etc) |
| | | | | 1 pint** | 0-12mo:breast/formula Under 2 y: full fat 2-5 y: semi-skimmed From 5 y: skimmed |

\* have 5 portions of fruit and vegetables per day at least
\*\* 1 pint = 3 x 150 g yogurts or 3 oz cheese

**Figure 10.14** The analysis sheet on which the details of the dietary analysis are recorded as well as a summary of the advice to be given. (NME = non-milk extrinsic.)

• **General nutritional intake.** This section examines how well the patient fares in relation to the major food groups as listed in the 'Balance of good health' (Fig. 7.1). Again, look at the table from the public health aspect. For example, crisps are not an acceptable form of potato; tomato ketchup is not an acceptable vegetable; and jam is not an acceptable fruit intake. While fruit is better than fruit juice, fruit juice is better than orange cordial. Thus, some quality judgements are necessary.

Record the intakes for each day, average them over the 3 days, and compare these figures with the recommendations. Most of the recommendations are given in terms of the number of portions per day but it is usual to assess volume of milk intake. It should be obvious to you whether there appears to be adequate intakes of cereals, vegetables, fruits, dairy products, and scope for increasing consumption of groups such as cereals, fresh fruit, and vegetables.

You will now need to dovetail this information with that obtained in the top table. As you analysed the diet, you will have noted some of the patient's likes and dislikes. Does he/she drink milk? Whole fruit? Pasta? Sandwiches? Use the right-hand column to list tentative recommendations. You are now ready for the third stage.

## Giving advice

You will need a record to give to the patient to take away. The leaflet shown in Fig. 10.15 is an example. The first inside page gives general oral health advice, the second inside page provides space for you to write goals agreed with the patient, and the back page gives examples of suitable snack foods which can be useful in many circumstances (see following pages).

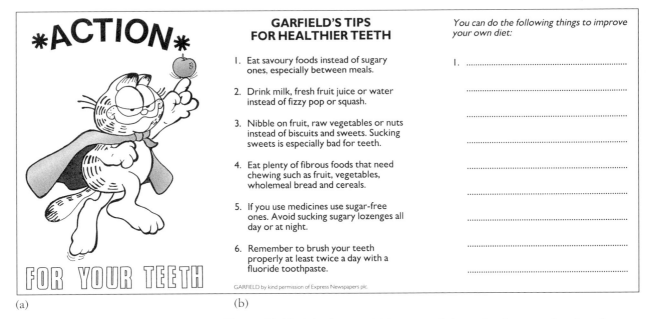

(a)　(b)

**Figure 10.15** A leaflet on which to record the patient's personal action plan as well as some general advice about dietary management: (a) outside front cover, (b) the inside pages. On the back cover is a list of suggestions for suitable snack foods and drinks (see Box 10.10).

Often, it is useful to begin by thanking the patient for taking the trouble to complete the dietary record; you have analysed it carefully and have some points to discuss. Always try to give some praise first. This is particularly true for parents, who are usually very proud of the way they are trying to bring up their children; initial criticism will deflate their self-esteem. Always accentuate the positive if at all possible.

It is sensible to discuss dietary aspects which are easiest to understand first. In this category will come the concept of avoiding sugary foods within an hour of bedtime. Most patients and parents will be able to understand this and it is also one of the easiest changes to make.

The importance of meals and the dangers of snacking with sugary foods and drinks are also concepts relatively easy to understand. However, changing from being a snacker to being a meal-eater may be quite difficult in practice, depending on the circumstances that surround regular eating, shopping, and cooking arrangements. Nevertheless, it is definitely worth discussing with the patient to see if there is any way to encourage preparation and consumption of meals rather than eating a succession of snacks. Your analysis of the general properties of the diet will be useful in advising on the better choices of foods for meals and snacks.

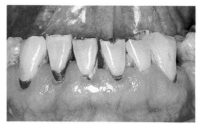

**Figure 10.16** An intraoral view of an elderly patient with extensive root caries. Reproduced with permission of Professor AWG Walls.

## Case report

Mr Boyles, a retired but active gentleman, lives on his own since becoming a widower 5 years ago. Like many men of his generation he has no cooking skills and is inclined to live out of a tin. Now that he is less active, his appetite has diminished and it is often easier to eat only biscuits and drink tea. Family members nearby give him a meal when he is babysitting for them, but they are busy with a young family so that does not happen often. 'Meals on wheels' is another alternative but he feels he is 'too young for that'. A complication is that his medication leaves him with a dry mouth, for which he tries to compensate by sucking lemon sweets, with the expected dental result (Fig. 10.16).

Mr Boyles needs advice on a healthier approach to his eating generally and specific help with his dry mouth. Mr Boyles has a microwave so that ready prepared meals can be defrosted and reheated, giving him a more balanced diet. He may then be less reliant on snacks, or if they are to remain a feature of his diet, then suggestions for safer alternatives are needed: toast with Marmite, sandwiches with low-fat spread, fruit, teacakes, bagels, and so on. As for the dry mouth, a prescription for a saliva substitute may be necessary although advice as given in Chapter 8 should be helpful. Sugar-free sweets in moderation may be the only change required.

Mr Boyles has grandchildren and it is important to stress also his responsibility when he is looking after them (Fig. 10.17); giving his grandchildren sweets and biscuits would be all too easy, but emphasizing the importance of their oral health as well as his own may avoid bad habits becoming established. He has to set the example.

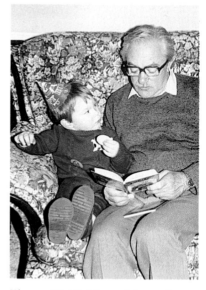

**Figure 10.17** Many older patients have a role in caring for grandchildren and thus have a responsibility for their diet too.

Sometimes the task of changing from being a snacker to being a meal-eater will be too great for the patient. Accept this and see whether there is scope for

## Box 10.10 **Snack foods and drinks for children**

(This list could go on the back page of the leaflet shown in Fig. 10.15.)

- Sandwich filled with salad, cheese spread, peanut butter, Marmite, Bovril, ham, cheese
- Crackers and cheese, pizza fingers, quiche fingers or tartlets, bread sticks
- Apple slices, orange segments, grapes, small banana, cherry tomatoes
- Yoghurt, unsweetened cereal with milk, milkshake, *fromage frais*
- Milk, water, well-diluted sugar-free squash*

* Not for infants if they contain non-sugar sweeteners.

## Box 10.11 **Summary points concerning a dietary record**

- The *patient* has a diet-related oral problem; *you* have the expert knowledge to help them.
- The patient will need much commitment to complete the dietary diary.
- Get all three appointments close together with only a week or so between each of the three stages.
- Don't give advice before stage 3.
- Advice should be *personal*, *practical*, and *positive*.

substituting poor quality (high-sugar, high-fat, high-salt) snacks for better quality snacks (high complex carbohydrate, fruit, and some forms of vegetables). If the choice of suitable snack foods seems difficult, turn to the back page of the leaflet and see if you can agree some of these with the patient. Talk through possibilities with the patient using examples of good practice from their own record. If the patient drank some milk during the 3 days, they cannot hate milk or be allergic to it. Thus, you may encourage milk consumption in place of other soft drinks, at least on some occasions.

The objective of these discussions is to agree a number of goals which the patient believes can be achieved. There should be no more than three, if they are to be remembered and acted upon. Include one that should be easy to achieve, and one or two that are 'dentally' important; it is far better to achieve some goals than to fail by being too ambitious. The achievable goals should be written down in the leaflet in the space provided on the second inside page. To an extent, this is the patient's contract with you—you are there to give him or her support and guidance to achieve these goals. End as you started, by trying to accentuate the positive. Do remember to have a dialogue, not a monologue from you. Encourage the patient to ask questions or make comments and listen to them. Lastly, but not least, your advice has to be *personal*, *practical*, and *positive*.

### Encouragement and reinforcement

Dietary change is difficult—encouragement and reinforcement of advice are essential. This is why you should write down the advice you agree with the patient on the diet analysis form. On the patient's next visit, you will then be well placed to ask about progress in making these changes. The 'contract' may have to be changed—that's fine, as long they are achievable goals which will improve health.

## Box 10.12 **Athletes**

Optimal fitness needs good nutrition. The energy needs of athletes are increased, often greatly if very heavy training and competitive sports are involved. Athletes are often the targets of those marketing questionable nutritive substances which are often suggested for use as ergogenic aids to increase performance. Perhaps the most worrying habits are the constant intake of sugars, especially as drinks; the missing of meals and their substitution by snacks; and the intermittent consumption of carbonated 'sports' drinks when dehydrated risking dental erosion. Intake of water and minerals is generally more important than intake of sugars, although much depends on the event and the level of performance. Athletes tend to put training and performance before any other consideration. There is a growing number of sports nutritionists who will be prepared to discuss advice with you. The use of anabolic steroids among adolescents to increase lean body mass and improve muscle strength is extremely dangerous from the health viewpoint: it may impair normal sexual function and stunt growth if it is used before maturity is attained.

# Handling problems

Some people will have dietary problems which are outside your level of expertise and these should be discussed with the patient's general medical practitioner (with the patient's permission) or refer the patient to a state registered dietitian. Patients on special diets or with difficult home circumstances were discussed earlier.

Sometimes you will find it difficult to believe the contents of the diet record. There may either be large gaps in the day's record or the record may be 'too good to be true'. In the former case, question gently about what the patient did during this 'empty time'. It is much better to accept the diet record as it is and use it as a vehicle for discussion. If the diet looks perfect—say how pleased you are to see this and discuss why you believe this to be good and the dangers of diets which were not like this one. In this way, the patient's record will become a useful vehicle for education.

Changing behaviour is often difficult. A patient may say 'I want to do what you say but I just can't manage'. Advice will not be sufficient and, if it is important to change behaviour, the patient may be referred for professional counselling. Such cases are beyond the dental practitioner's area of expertise.

## Box 10.13  **Using dietitians**

You will be competent to give dietary advice to the vast majority of your patients. There are three occasions when it would be sensible to seek further advice:
- when patients are on special diets
- when you discover bizarre eating habits
- when you are unlikely to achieve dietary change because of the patient's home circumstances.

In these cases, the patient should be referred to a dietitian. The term 'dietitian' is not protected and in the UK anyone may call themselves a dietitian. Only state registered dietitians are registered with the Council for Professions Supplementary to Medicine and hence possess approved qualifications and are subject to its code of conduct. This code binds dietitians only to accept referrals from medical practitioners or dental practitioners and only state registered dietitians are currently employed by the NHS.

Most large hospitals employ dietitians but their workloads concern mainly therapeutic diets, although many will accept outpatient referrals for dietary appraisal only. Many districts employ community dietitians whose remit is to take dietetic services into the local communities. This may involve setting up regular clinics in health centres which could be more convenient for patients referred for assessment and advice. Health promotion units too may employ dietitians who are less likely to be willing to carry out individual appraisals but could provide much valuable general support (information, equipment, and advice) to the practitioner. It is therefore highly desirable for dental practitioners to establish exactly what service is available to them from their local dietitians.

# How effective is dietary advice?

Dietary treatment of a wide variety of disorders can save and prolong lives and reduce morbidity. There is little doubt that therapeutic diets are effective if changes in habits take place. Where life-threatening disorders are concerned, motivation and hence compliance can be high, but studies of adherence with weight-reducing diets generally indicate a rather poor success rate. Even adherence with diabetic diets is generally poor, but individuals do comply as well as they are able or as well as their circumstances will allow. A hundred per cent adherence with any advice should not be expected and any changes achieved should be regarded as 'success'. It is vital to convince patients that they want to change their habits and to negotiate these changes in order to achieve success. The dietary record forms an excellent basis for these discussions.

## Case report

Paul is a child of a mixed marriage whose parents are separated. He is now 10 years old and shares his time between two households. When he was first seen in the surgery he was nearly 5 years old and with an apparently caries-free dentition (Figs 10.18 and 10.19). Bitewing radiographs taken then revealed approximal lesions in his primary molars. Since that time, he has followed a stricter dietary regime, used fluoride toothpaste, a daily 0.05 per cent sodium fluoride mouthwash, and had fluoride varnish applied approximally with floss, 4 monthly on dental visits, as well as sealants to his first permanent molar teeth on eruption. His diet record 6 months ago reflects sensible eating for a 10 year old, with between one and three intakes per day of non-milk extrinsic sugars (Fig. 10.22). Radiographs show, compared with the baseline views when Paul was nearly 5 years old, and views taken at 10 years of age, that these lucencies have not increased and may even have remineralized in the case of tooth 84 (Figs 10.20 and 10.21).

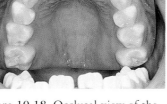

**Figure** 10.18 Occlusal view of the upper arch of the child, 5 years after the instigation of dietary advice. There is no evidence of cavitated lesions.

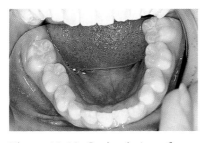

**Figure** 10.19 Occlusal view of the lower arch of the patient in Fig. 10.18.

This case points out the necessity of taking a good history as well as baseline records. Having identified caries at this first occasion, aggressive prevention was the key to success. Whilst you might assume that a clinically caries-free dentition indicates a healthy mouth, bitewing radiographs at this stage can be humbling: caries is into dentine and prevention alone will not be the answer.

Social circumstances have changed to the extent that the nuclear family as we understood it—two parents married to each other with two children—is no longer the norm. With child patients of split families, there is the opportunity for one parent to 'blame' the other for dietary indiscretions and the child may even play off one side of the family against the other. Parents may compensate for their guilt by giving in to the child or children and allowing confectionery and fizzy drinks to be consumed frequently, in order to win favour with their offspring. You need to be sensitive to these issues and work around them.

There have been far too few studies of the effectiveness of dietary advice specifically in relation to dental caries or dental erosion. Reductions in decay of 40–65 per cent have been observed to result from dietary advice based on only three sessions. There can be no doubt that advice to reduce the intake of sugars is

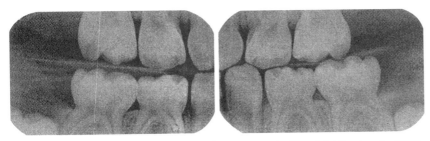

**Figure 10.20** Bitewing radiographs of the patient in Fig. 10.18 taken in 1992.

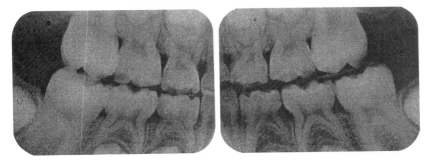

**Figure 10.21** Bitewing radiographs of the patient in Fig. 10.18 taken in 1997 showing little progression of enamel lucencies 5 years later.

**Figure 10.22** A page from the 1997 3 day dietary record of the child in Fig. 10.18.

safe, timely, and effective and, in addition, each patient is entitled to the most comprehensive advice possible.

Changing dietary habits to improve health is not easy. The many powerful pressures working against health were discussed in the previous chapters. It is important to realize that dietary habits do change, and that it is the task of health professionals to encourage them to change in the right direction.

## Summary

- Many factors influence people's dietary habits, for example, physiological, psychological, economic and cultural needs.

- Establish relevant aspects of the patient's history first, for example, medical and social factors.

- All patients should receive general dietary advice; patients with specific needs may require a more detailed dietary investigation.

- Allow time for the dietary record to be completed, analysed and discussed with the patient.

- Work at establishing a partnership between you and the patient in order to achieve changes in behaviour.

- Be aware of, and use, other resources, for example, community dietitians, where the patient's needs are beyond the sphere of your expertise.

- Throughout, make what you have to say **personal**, **practical** and **positive**.

## Further reading

British Postgraduate Medical Federation (1990). *Sweetness and light. A practical guide to giving advice on sugar, diet and dental health*. A video produced by the British Postgraduate Medical Federation, London.

Health Education Authority (1993). *Changing what you eat. A guide for primary health care workers*. Health Education Authority, London.

Niven, N. (1994). *Health psychology* (2nd edn), Chapters 1–3, 6. Churchill Livingstone, Edinburgh.

Rugg-Gunn, A. J. *Nutrition and dental health*, Chapter 16. Oxford University Press, Oxford.

# To close

Diet and nutrition grab the headlines almost every day—we are quite obsessed by what we eat and what our food does or does not do for us—but it is a topic that has gained prominence in the last decade. We now have a plethora of reports pertaining to healthy eating, a Food Standards Agency, professors of psychiatry to manage patients with eating disorders and a growing problem of malnutrition in the western world—that of obesity.

What of oral health in all this? The link between sugars in the diet and poor dental health is as strong as ever, related perhaps now more to deprivation. Since Nutrition and Dental Health was written, the evidence linking what we consume to erosion of teeth has become more compelling, and we are more confident of the relationship between protective factors in foods and oral cancer.

This would be a dismal list if it were to stop there, but there is much to applaud in the way of progress: government endorsement of moves to encourage eating for health, successful health promotion campaigns, manufacturers slowly responding to consumer and professional pressure for a change to healthy options, and a growing awareness that we are what we eat. In the midst of change, the dental team have a professional responsibility—ethical and legal—to be informed in what they say to, and do for, patients. Managing a patient's oral health—preventing the preventable—is the fundamental right of all patients and the duty of the dentist. Appropriate, informed dietary advice is the corner-stone of a successful preventive practice, in a partnership involving the patient, the professional and, more recently, industry and government.

# Index